Practical Prescribing for Medical Students

Titles in the Series

Health, Behaviour and Society: Clinical Medicine in Context ISBN 9780857254610
Innovating for Patient Safety in Medical Practice ISBN 9780857257659
Practical Prescribing for Medical Students ISBN 9781446256398
Professional Practice for Foundation Doctors ISBN 9780857252845
Succeeding in Your Medical Degree ISBN 9780857253972

You can find more information on each of these titles and our other learning resources at www.sagepub.co.uk

Practical Prescribing for Medical Students

Editors:

Helen Bradbury and Barry Strickland-Hodge

Series Editors:

Judy McKimm and Kirsty Forrest

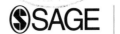

Los Angeles | London | New Delhi
Singapore | Washington DC

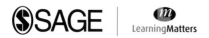

Learning Matters
An imprint of SAGE Publications Ltd
1 Oliver's Yard
55 City Road
London EC1Y 1SP

SAGE Publications Inc.
2455 Teller Road
Thousand Oaks, California 91320

SAGE Publications India Pvt Ltd
B 1/I 1 Mohan Cooperative Industrial Area
Mathura Road
New Delhi 110 044

SAGE Publications Asia-Pacific Pte Ltd
3 Church Street
#10-04 Samsung Hub
Singapore 049483

Editor: Alex Clabburn
Development editor: Richenda Milton-Daws
Production controller: Chris Marke
Project management: Swales & Willis Ltd,
Exeter, Devon
Marketing manager: Tamara Navaratnam
Cover design: Wendy Scott
Typeset by: C&M Digitals (P) Ltd, Chennai, India
Printed by: Henry Ling Limited at The Dorset
Press, Dorchester, DT1 1HD

**Library of Congress Control Number:
2013947941**

**British Library Cataloguing in Publication
data**

A catalogue record for this book is available
from the British Library

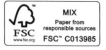

ISBN 978-1-4462-5639-8
ISBN 978-1-4462-5640-4 (pbk)

Contents

Foreword from the Series Editors

The Learning Matters Medical Education Series

Medical education is currently experiencing yet another a period of change, typified in the UK with the introduction of the revised *Tomorrow's Doctors* (General Medical Council, 2009) and ongoing work on establishing core curricula for many subject areas. Changes are also occurring at Foundation and postgraduate levels in terms of the introduction of broader non-technical competencies, a wider range of assessments and new revalidation requirements. This new series of textbooks has been developed as a direct response to these changes and the impact on all levels of medical education.

Research indicates that effective medical practitioners combine excellent, up-to-date clinical and scientific knowledge with practical skills and the ability to work with patients, families and other professionals with empathy and understanding; they know when to lead and when to follow and they work collaboratively and professionally to improve health outcomes for individuals and communities. In *Tomorrow's Doctors*, the General Medical Council defines a series of learning outcomes set out under three headings:

1. Doctor as Practitioner;
2. Doctor as Scholar and Scientist;
3. Doctor as Professional.

The books in this series do not cover practical clinical procedures or knowledge about diseases and conditions, but instead cover the range of non-technical professional skills (plus underpinning knowledge) that students and doctors need to know in order to become effective, safe and competent practitioners.

Aimed specifically at medical students (but also of use for junior doctors, teachers and clinicians), each book relates to specific outcomes of *Tomorrow's Doctors* and other relevant documents, providing both knowledge and help to improve the skills necessary to be successful at the non-clinical aspects of training as a doctor. One of the aims of the series is to set medical practice within wider social, policy and organisational agendas to help produce future doctors who are socially aware and willing and prepared to engage in broader issues relating to healthcare delivery.

Individual books in the series outline the key theoretical approaches and policy agendas relevant to that subject, and go further by demonstrating through case studies and scenarios how these theories can be used in work settings to achieve best practice. Plenty of activities and self-assessment tools throughout the book will help readers to hone their critical thinking and reflection skills.

Chapters in each of the books follow a standard format. At the beginning a box highlights links to relevant competencies and outcomes from *Tomorrow's Doctors* and other curricula, if appropriate. This sets the scene and enables readers to see exactly what will be covered. This is extended by a chapter overview which sets out the key topics and learning outcomes.

Each chapter typically includes at least one case study which illustrates how theory can be used in practice from different perspectives. Activities are included which include practical tasks with learning points, critical thinking research tasks and reflective practice/thinking points. Activities can be carried out by readers or with others and are designed to raise awareness, consolidate understanding and enable students to improve their practice by using models, approaches and ideas. Each activity is followed by a brief discussion on issues raised. At the end of each chapter a chapter summary provides an aide-mémoire of what has been covered.

All chapters are evidence-based in that they set out the theories or evidence that underpins practice. In most chapters, one or more 'What's the evidence?' boxes provide further information about a particular piece of research or a policy agenda referenced in books, articles, websites or policy papers. A list of additional readings is set out under the 'Going further' section, with all references collated at the end of the book.

The series is edited by Professor Judy McKimm and Professor Kirsty Forrest, both of whom are experienced medical educators and writers. Book and chapter authors are drawn from a wide pool of practising clinicians and educators from around the world.

Author Biographies

David Alldred, formerly of the University of Leeds, now Senior Lecturer in Pharmacy Practice at the School of Pharmacy, University of Bradford. David is a clinical pharmacist who has research and practice experience in primary and secondary care. His teaching and research focus on the quality and safe use of medicines, particularly in older people.

Helen Bradbury, Senior Lecturer at the University of Leeds. Helen's post at Leeds spans education and healthcare. She is the programme leader for the Master's in Clinical Education and has published on reflective practice and e-learning. Helen worked in the NHS for 20 years as a hospital pharmacist before commencing her academic career.

Natalie Bryars, Principal Pharmacist at York Teaching Hospital NHS Foundation Trust, where she leads on Clinical Governance. Natalie's teaching focuses on medicines management and patient safety and she contributes to the training programmes for medical, nursing and pharmacy staff within the Trust. She also teaches on prescribing at the Hull and York Medical School and her research has focused on how prescribing can be taught more effectively to medical students.

Catherine Gill, Lecturer and Module Leader Nurse Prescribing, University of Leeds, Lead Partner for Learning and Teaching, Caritas Health Partnership. Catherine has a keen interest in prescribing and holistic practice and was among the first UK nurses to qualify as an independent nurse prescriber. Since then she has combined clinical practice with academia, promoting interprofessional learning and teaching and achieving appointment as an associate GP trainer.

Daniel Greer, Lead Pharmacist for Gastroenterology, Leeds Teaching Hospitals NHS Trust. Daniel's background is in hospital pharmacy, where he has worked since qualifying as a pharmacist in 1994. He joined the University of Leeds as a lecturer practitioner and helped set up a new postgraduate programme in pharmacy practice. He contributes to other pharmacology and therapeutics teaching within the school and wider university as well as supervising MSc student dissertations.

Greg Heath, Specialty Registrar in Medical Ophthalmology, York Teaching Hospital NHS Foundation Trust. Greg has an active role in teaching undergraduate and postgraduate students in medicine. He also lectures optometrists on independent prescribing at City University, London.

Andy Hutchinson, Medicines Education Technical Adviser, Medicines and Prescribing Centre at the National Institute for Health and Care Excellence (NICE). Andy is a pharmacist who has been teaching doctors, pharmacists and nurses about evidence-based medicine for more than 20 years. He is particularly interested in the practical skills that busy health professionals need to make evidence-informed decisions with their patients.

Monica Murphy, Student Education Fellow and Lecturer in Ethics and Law in the School of Healthcare, University of Leeds. Monica is a nurse prescriber with a special interest in adult safeguarding and developing student education on medicines management.

Barry Strickland-Hodge, Director, Academic Unit of Pharmacy, Radiography and Healthcare Science and Senior Pharmacy Lecturer, School of Healthcare, University of Leeds. Barry is a pharmacist and information scientist leading on independent prescribing for pharmacists. He teaches nurses, midwives, radiographers, pharmacists, psychiatrists and medical students. As an apothecary, he also has an interest in the history of pharmacy and medicine.

Jonathan Underhill, Associate Director Medicines Evidence, Medicines and Prescribing Centre at the National Institute for Health and Care Excellence (NICE). Jonathan is a pharmacist with a background in medicines evaluation, education and advice. He is passionate about the practical application of the science and art of evidence-informed decision making to help practitioners ensure the best possible outcomes for their patients.

Arnold Zermansky, retired general practitioner and Honorary Senior Research Fellow in the School of Healthcare, University of Leeds. Arnold's teaching and research focus on the quality and safe use of medicines.

Abbreviations

ACE	angiotensin-converting enzyme
ADE	adverse drug event
ADR	adverse drug reaction
APTT	activated partial thromboplastin time
BNF	*British National Formulary*
BNF-C	*BNF for Children*
CD	controlled drug
CI	confidence interval
CNS	central nervous system
CrCL	creatinine clearance
DAP	drug analysis print
EBM	evidence-based medicine
ECG	electrocardiogram
FSRH	Faculty of Sexual and Reproductive Healthcare
GFR	glomerular filtration rate
GMC	General Medical Council
GSL	general sales list
ICE	ideas, concerns and expectations
INR	international normalised ratio
IV	intravenous
LMWH	low-molecular-weight heparin
MA	marketing authorisation
MAOI	monoamine oxidase inhibitor
MDRD	modification of diet in renal disease
MHRA	Medicines and Healthcare Products Regulatory Agency
NHS	National Health Service
NHS IQ	NHS Improving Quality
NICE	National Institute for Health and Care Excellence
NKDA	no known drug allergies
NNH	number needed to harm
NNT	number needed to treat
NPC	National Prescribing Centre
NPSA	National Patient Safety Agency
NSAID	non-steroidal anti-inflammatory drug
OTC	over the counter
P	pharmacy medicines
PGD	Patient Group Direction
P-gp	P-glycoprotein
POM	prescription-only medicine
PSD	Patient Specific Direction
RCT	randomised controlled trial
SIGN	Scottish Intercollegiate Guidelines Network
SPC	Summary of Product Characteristics

Introduction: The Challenge of Prescribing

Arnold Zermansky

This introduction is to whet your appetite to the challenge of prescribing and alert you to its complexity and human dimension.

> *To write prescriptions is easy, but to come to an understanding with people is hard.*

(Kafka, 1983, p. 223)

Kafka's much-quoted aphorism is naive in two respects. First, it understates the challenge of prescribing. Second, it implies that prescribing is a mere technical skill that does not require the meeting of minds between prescriber and patient that is vital to all clinical encounters. This book will demonstrate the need for skill in prescribing. It will also show how interpersonal skills are as important as technical knowledge if prescribing is to be effective and safe.

What is prescribing for?

At its simplest, prescribing is a mechanism for ensuring that a patient is dispensed the medicine that the prescriber requires. The purist might point out that (especially in UK general practice) prescriptions can be for dressings, appliances and other non-pharmaceuticals, but for simplicity I exclude these from this discussion. This mechanical definition seriously understates the complexity of the process and excludes the patient from an active role. A better definition would start with the agreed formulation of the patient's problem or problems, work through the natural history of the problems identified, consider the risks and benefits of pharmaceutical intervention, choose the most appropriate treatment (if any) and only then decide how to ensure that the patient receives it in the safest, most effective and efficient way. The participants in the process must at the very least include the treating clinician, patient and dispensing pharmacist, but may also include other clinicians caring for the patient, the patient's relatives and carers, pathologist, nurse, practice receptionist, dispensing technician, and even the neighbour who collects the medicine from the pharmacist.

Is this sort of inclusivity really important in the prescribing process? Does the doctor with fingers poised above the prescribing keyboard really need to think about all this? Or is this just another example of the 'politically correct thought police' complicating everything we do?

Think of a patient, Mrs Wellstone, who is aged 87. She lives alone in her supported flat. She is attended twice daily by professional carers (who are employed by an agency on behalf of Social Services). She takes lots of tablets for her heart condition, including a statin and warfarin. These are supplied by the local pharmacy in a monitored-dosage box.

Mrs Wellstone has become more confused this week and her daughter calls the doctor. She has a temperature of 37.8°C, a rattling cough, but no definite signs in the chest. The patient cannot easily provide a urine specimen as she is incontinent. The doctor suspects a chest infection but cannot exclude the possibility of a urinary infection and is minded to prescribe an antibiotic. 'She doesn't want to go back in hospital again after the last time', says the daughter.

Think about the constraints and pressures (overt or unstated) that should influence Mrs Wellstone's prescriber in arriving at a prescribing plan. In doing so consider the pharmacology but also practical, pragmatic, patient-centred and professional issues.

You know that she is too unwell to wait until a specimen has been obtained before prescribing. If hospital admission is to be avoided it is important to choose an antibiotic which is likely to show rapid results for both diagnoses. Remember that 50% of community-acquired urinary tract infections are resistant to amoxicillin. You know that she is on several tablets, including a statin and warfarin, that may interact adversely with some antibiotics.

The Health Protection Agency advises against prescribing cephalosporins as first-line agents because of the risk of increasing *Clostridium difficile* infections. As Mrs Wellstone is confused, the choice of antibiotic requires that taking the drug will have to be prompted by the carers, who only visit twice a day, so medication should be chosen which only needs to be given twice a day.

Which can we choose?

Amoxicillin would be a satisfactory choice for a chest infection, but not for a urinary tract infection. Macrolide antibiotics are especially likely to enhance the anticoagulant effect of warfarin which we know she is taking. Quinolone antibiotics are commonly ineffective against pneumococci.

It may be appropriate to put the patient's need above the risk to the community and prescribe a cephalosporin. The patient's carers and daughter will need to be included in the care plan to ensure that the medicines are taken properly.

Follow-up to ensure that the patient improves promptly is vital, and may require a further visit, by either the GP or another team member.

Finally the GP may need to consider whether admission to hospital rather than prescription might be the safest option. This would require persuading the patient and her daughter of the advisability of this option.

This all goes to highlight the decision-making tree that needs to be followed for what might appear to be a simple case of infection in an elderly woman.

The purpose of this complex case study is to demonstrate that very complexity. Prescribing is not just a simple mechanical task. Anything involving people is inherently complicated and needs careful consideration.

The ramifications of your prescribing may be finite, but not always visible.

Throughout this book you will come across examples of drug interactions (Chapter 9), adverse drug reactions (Chapter 8), errors in prescribing (Chapter 7) as well as how to communicate with patients (Chapter 1) in order to ensure you have all the information you need to make decisions. You can prescribe the correct drug at the correct dose for the correct time and yet the patient may decide not to take the drug or to take someone else's. By reading this book you will see how a concordant relationship with a patient can help to minimise such problems.

People and their pills

Repeat prescriptions are written in steel and concrete and are not easily dismantled or remodelled.

(Balint *et al.*, 1970)

At least 75% of GP prescription items are for long-term treatment (Harris and Dajda, 1996). These are medicines that are taken (or are meant to be taken) for months or years or even decades. The actual numbers of medicines prescribed in the community are staggering. In 2011 for England alone there were 961 million prescription items dispensed at a net ingredient cost of £8.8 billion (NHS Information Centre, 2012). Repeats are generally for the control of long-term conditions such as diabetes, asthma or epilepsy, or for the prevention of disease or its complications. The growth in preventive prescribing in the last decade or so has been fuelled in part by the emergence of sound evidence for the value of such interventions, in part by the systemisation of risk assessment and in part by the development and marketing of effective and safer drugs. GPs have become better at identifying and actively pursuing patients with chronic conditions, thereby ensuring that patients live longer and in consequence continue to take their medicines for longer, which further increases the rate of repeat prescribing.

There is, of course a different level of gearing for preventive interventions than for acute therapy. While one would hope that the number needed to treat (NNT) for short-term important illnesses such as pneumonia would be close to one, the same is not true for hypertension or cholesterol-lowering treatment, where NNT may be in the hundreds and needs to be calculated over years rather than days or weeks. This in turn has a major implication in terms of the benefit-to-harm ratio (see Chapter 3 for a more detailed discussion). While the likelihood of a patient benefiting from, say, a treatment for hypertension may be less than 1% per annum (Bandolier, 1997), the risk of adverse effects from a hypertensive drug is not likely to be less than that of any other drug. So more patients are likely to be harmed by the drug than benefit from it. If this is true, why do we ever prescribe preventive medicines?

Finding a definitive answer to the simple question, 'What are the benefits and risks of the drug treatment of moderate hypertension?' is surprisingly difficult. The possible combinations of patient age and sex, drug choice and baseline level of blood pressure are almost infinite. Bandolier's table gives a flavour of this diversity (see Bandolier, 1997).

I hope you will have recognised that, for the individual patient, taking a repeat medication is an article of faith. The patient who swallows the pill has to share the prescriber's view of the value of the medicine. This is particularly so in the case of a preventive medicine, because the best the patient can expect to happen is nothing. If the medicine works, the patient will not develop the symptoms of the illness. And, with luck, he/she will not experience any adverse effects. So the patient will be taking a tablet (or maybe several) every day for years with no discernible effect.

Compliance, adherence and concordance are addressed in Chapter 1. These issues probably make up the most challenging dimension of prescribing because it encompasses all facets of human behaviour in patient and (less obviously) prescriber, dispenser and carer. Knowledge of pharmacology does not prepare you for this vital area.

People get attached to their medicines. They develop rituals and belief systems around them. For reasons that are emotional and psychological as well as pharmacological, the medicines become an integral part of their daily lives. But patients change, their illnesses change, the science of therapeutics changes. The medicine that is ideal and appropriate now may cease to be so in the future. It is therefore vital to review patients' medicines and their need for them at appropriate intervals. You will probably know that GP practices and pharmacies and care homes have developed complex computer systems to control and manage repeat medication but these are seldom in tandem, unfortunately. When you visit a general practice or a pharmacy (and you would benefit from visiting both), take the opportunity to look at the system and how it works. Observe the skills of the receptionists and dispensing assistants. Consider the strengths and weaknesses of the systems.

Having now explored the bigger picture, perhaps now is the time to get down to the process of prescribing and see how we should go about it. You obviously need a pen to sign the prescription and a piece of paper to write (or print) on. It would help to have a formulary like the *British National Formulary* (BNF, 2013), which is available online and as an App. It contains a lot more than the doses of drugs. And you also need a patient with a condition. The BNF will be referred to throughout this book, so get a copy or have access to it.

Decades ago, as a medical student, I learned several painful lessons from one unfortunate incident. At that time medical students who performed as locums for house officers (now FY1s) were allowed to prescribe. I was a locum for the orthopaedic house officer and tagged along on the registrar's ward round. We came to the bed of a young man who had osteomyelitis and the registrar told me to prescribe for him an antibiotic called Cristamycin. I duly did as I was told and prescribed the drug by 6-hourly intramuscular injection. Fortunately the patient never received his first injection. I knew he was allergic to penicillin but thought I was prescribing a brand of streptomycin (an aminoglycoside antibiotic). What I didn't know, because I did not look it up, was that Cristamycin contained benzyl penicillin as well as streptomycin. It was the ward sister who intervened to prevent the patient getting the drug, and it was she who bore down on me like a battleship at full speed with guns blazing. I deserved all I got, and I learned four vital lessons:

1. Medicines have a capacity for harm as well as for good – and so do prescribers.

2. Obeying orders is no excuse for getting your prescription wrong. It is always the signatory who is responsible, both morally and legally.

3. Your profession is not the sole custodian of wisdom. You can and should learn from professionals in other disciplines and from your patients. Ignore them at your peril.

4. Humility is not the opposite of self-confidence. It is actually part of it.

Some common calculations are shown in Appendix 1, with the answers following. In the spirit of learning, perhaps it would be wise to try the calculations first, and then check you have them right.

The regulation and law, how to prescribe, when to do it (and when not to) will become clearer as you read on. This is information you need to know to be effective and safe. My hope for you is that you use it as a launching pad for effective, safe, intelligent and, where appropriate, creative prescribing.

And finally, this book has been written by medical doctors, academic pharmacists and nurses. And in the words of Rabbi Ben Zoma:

Who is wise? One who learns from everyone, as it is said, 'From all my teachers I gained wisdom'.

(Rabbi Ben Zoma (2nd century), 2006)

chapter 1

Communication and Patient Collaboration

Catherine Gill and Monica Murphy

Achieving your medical degree

This chapter will help you begin to meet the following requirements of *Tomorrow's Doctors* (General Medical Council (GMC), 2009):

Outcome 2: The doctor as a practitioner

13. Carry out a consultation which elicits patients' questions, their understanding of their condition and treatment options, and their views, concerns, values and preferences: (a), (b), (f), (g).

15. Communicate effectively with patients and colleagues: (a), (b), (c), (f), (g), (h).

17. Prescribe drugs safely, effectively and economically: (a), (c), (d), (e), (f), (h).

It will also link to:

Good Medical Practice (GMC, 2013a)

and

Good Practice in Prescribing and Managing Medicines and Devices (GMC, 2013b), particularly paragraphs 14, 16, 21–24 and 25–29.

A Single Competency Framework for all Prescribers (National Prescribing Centre, 2012) 2:12, 21, 23, 24 3: 25-37, 4:45, 5:49, 8: 66, 9:70.

Chapter overview

This chapter provides an outline of the essential communication and consultation skills that you will need to master in order to achieve the minimum standard expected of a prescriber. The application of these skills will help you not only in the detective work involved in clinical supposition and differential diagnosis but also in choosing correct treatment options. In more cases than not, the treatment options you choose will involve the prescribing of medicines; and, as you will learn elsewhere in this book, can result in adverse effects for patients regardless of whether this was the correct treatment option. Research shows that if you gather quality information which includes the patient's concerns, ideas and expectations, and negotiate treatment and management options, and warn regarding possible unwanted drug effects, then the likelihood of you being able to help the patient is greatly increased (NICE, 2009).

After reading this chapter you will be able to:

- describe the different models of consultation;
- explain how using bio-psycho-social models which take account of cultural and existential dimensions can positively influence medicine-taking behaviours;
- distinguish between the concepts of compliance, adherence and concordance;
- discuss the attitudes, knowledge and communication skills involved in patient-centred practice;
- recognise how the application of these skills can help patients take medicines safely.

ACTIVITY 1.1 DECIDING WHAT COMMUNICATION IS

This may seem elementary, but think about communication and what it is. Write a short list of the key principles of effective communication. You will discover a discussion of these in this chapter. When you have finished reading the chapter, look back at what you have written and see how what has been discussed compares to your initial list.

In *Tomorrow's Doctors,* the GMC states: *Medicine involves personal interaction with people, as well as the application of science and technical skills* (GMC, 2009, p. 4). This statement may surprise you – that an apparent fundamental in the practice of medicine needs to be articulated. Except in circumstances where a patient is unconscious, the application of science and technical skills cannot occur in a vacuum and communication with the person who needs medical attention, and/or next of kin, is essential. It seems sensible that medical practice involves a tripartite process of good communication, reasoning skills arising from scientific knowledge and clinical abilities. In an earlier GMC Standards document, *Good Medical Practice,* there is reference to *the new world of partnership with patients and colleagues* (GMC, 2006, p. 6). This suggests that, in the old world of medicine prior to 2006, partnership with patients, often referred to as a good 'bedside manner', was considered desirable but not essential.

The idea that good communication can improve patient health outcomes is not new and in the last 30 years of the twentieth century a strong body of work emerged exploring the rich potential of holism in healthcare. Much of the research undertaken since, to substantiate or disprove the validity of a holistic approach, has demonstrated better outcomes for patients (Edlin and Golanty, 1992; Department of Health, 2005; UKCCC, 2006). What occurs during a patient and doctor/clinician interaction – the consultation (to seek counsel) – has been extensively studied and what constitutes a successful consultation according to the patient can vary from the viewpoint of the clinician.

The consultation can be understood as a problem-solving process. The problem is something that needs consideration by the clinician. Consideration is a thought process of analysis and discernment (diagnostic process), with the endpoint being a judgement (diagnosis).

The remit of this chapter is to help you develop communication skills that will enable you to undertake a holistic consultation which is efficient and effective, yet caring and well rounded (Pietroni, 1987). The technicalities and reasoning skills related to thorough information gathering and information sharing are covered extensively, with little reference to the review of the biophysical systems and the physical examination, since these aspects are commonly covered in other medical texts.

What components make up an effective consultation?

Efficient and thorough information gathering influences the precision of diagnosis and therefore treatment by 80%. Studies repeatedly indicate this; however, patients think it is the opposite – that the laying on of hands (examination) is the most influential, along with investigations such as blood tests and X-rays/scans. The success of the consultation hinges on clinical knowledge and interview/planning skills and on the nature of the relationship that exists between clinician and patient. Your behaviour and attitude are just as important as what you say (Gray and Toghill, 2000; Bub, 2004; Deveugele *et al.*, 2004).

What is communication?

According to the *Oxford Dictionary* (2012), communication can be defined in a number of ways, but for the purposes of this chapter it is:

- the exchange of information, between people by means of speaking, writing or using a common system of signs and behaviours;
- a spoken or written message;
- rapport: a sense of mutual understanding and sympathy.

The patient needs to feel sufficiently confident in your abilities, and this perception may be based on your behaviour as observed by the patient: how you greet, whether you smile, do you present as rushed or stressed? Do you seek permission on how to address the patient – given name, title and family name? Once in the consultation room or by the bedside, your opening gambit can influence first impressions. How you invite patients to disclose their problem(s) is fairly influential (a number of useful opening phrases are listed in Table 1.1, below); what is more powerful, however, is how much time you give patients initially to explain what is worrying them. This is referred to as the 'golden minute'. Allowing patients to speak without interruption can give you almost all the information you need to unpick their problem. It also has the psychological benefit of helping patients to feel you understand them (Moutlon, 2007, p. 23). Given the quality of information you can gather from the patient perspective, their narrative and the patient-centredness that can be fostered, it would seem like time well spent. The urge to drill down with questioning to get to the bottom of the patient's problem, as you perceive it as the clinician, can be quite irresistible and may lead to premature and inaccurate assumptions.

> *A Patient is the most important person in our Hospital. He is not an interruption to our work. He is the purpose of it. He is not an outsider in our Hospital, he is part of it.*

> *We are not doing him a favour by serving him; he is doing us a favour by giving us an opportunity to do so.*

> (Bombay hospital motto, adapted from a quotation of Mahatma Gandhi)

ACTIVITY 1.2 HOW TO OPEN THE CONSULTATION

Before looking at Table 1.1 which details some useful opening phrases, put yourself in the position of a patient and think about what invitation phrase would induce you to share your problem(s) and what might turn you off.

If you have already adopted an opening phrase, what made you choose it?

How might age, gender and cultural background affect the opening phrase?

When is silence uncomfortable, and why?

Discuss your thoughts with a colleague and if possible a more experienced clinician. See if there are similarities and/or differences.

Table 1.1 Opening questions for the consultation

The following phrases are useful to invite patients to disclose their problem(s) and begin their narrative. They can be used after greeting the patient and introducing yourself. Whichever you use will be dependent on the healthcare setting; all can be used in general practice settings whereas questions 4–9 are more suitable for the hospital setting:

1. 'How can I help you today?'
2. 'What can I do for you today?'
3. 'What would you like to discuss with me?'
4. 'What has been happening to bring you here today?'
5. 'Would you like to tell me what's been going on?'
6. 'Tell me a little about why you have come today.'
7. 'If you'd like to tell me all about what's bothering you; when did it start?'
8. 'Could you start at the beginning and tell me how this all began?'
9. 'What has brought you here today?'

Non-verbal communication

In the general practice setting, opening/inviting phrases can actually distract from what the patient may have rehearsed to say and the use of silence with non-verbal communication following greeting and introductions can be more effective. These are referred to as non-verbal cues and involve active listening. Active listening includes observable behaviours of smiling, making and then maintaining eye contact, nodding and using facial expressions that indicate interest and understanding on your part. Other non-verbal communications that create or represent meaning are your body movements and gestures, often known under the mnemonic SOLER: sitting *square* on to the patient with an *open* position, *leaning* slightly forward with *eye* contact in a *relaxed* posture (Power, 1998) all imply a more interested and caring attitude.

Take care when using verbal expressions such as 'OK' as this can potentially present as impatience rather than interest. Better verbal encouragers include 'I see'; 'ah-ha'; 'yes'; 'go on'; 'uh-huh'; 'umm'.

Other lines of enquiry and exploration

When patients have fully exhausted what they have to say, you should then ask, 'Is there anything else?' This process is known as screening and can be used a number of times in the information-gathering stage. It is a deliberate method of checking back with patients regarding any other important symptoms and perceptions they may not have mentioned. You can now move the narrative thread on with open questions or open enquiry.

Open questions do not suggest an answer or bias the patient towards replying with what you would want in order to confirm your clinical conjecture. For example, posing a question such as, 'You're not breathless, are you?' may invite a 'no' response due to the bias; in fact, the patient may not be breathless at that moment but may have breathlessness at other times. A more appropriate open question is: 'Do you get breathless?'

It is not only important to listen to patients' initial narrative, but also to be able to direct patients once you have picked up the thread of the narrative. Essentially use open questions to direct and encourage patients to 'tell their story'. Some of these open questions may also be specific in order to clarify meaning and resolve ambiguity. Table 1.2 details a number of useful phrases to help you with open questions/enquiry and clarification. There is no hierarchy of importance; the golden minute is important and open questions are one of the most effective information-gathering tools.

Following exhaustion of your open questions, move to closed questions. You will need to have in mind a diagnosis or a number of potential diagnoses in order for you to ask closed questions to rule in or rule out. Closed questions enable you to test your clinical conjecture and 'fill in' any holes, which is ideal now but not before this stage.

Table 1.2 Developing information-gathering skills

The following phrases and techniques are useful to invite patients to expand on their problem(s) and their narrative.

Phrases

1. 'What did you mean when you said the drug 'upset' you?'
2. 'You mentioned earlier ... : can you tell me more about that?'
3. 'Could you explain what you mean by ... ?'
4. 'Please expand further on what you meant by ... '
5. 'I am interested in what you said earlier about ... : I would like to explore this a little more.'
6. 'Can you tell me a little more about what you said about ... ?'

Techniques

Reflecting (echoing) back statements, using vocal inflection which turns the patient's statement into a question and using hanging sentences or a single word followed by silence encourage expansion:

'you mentioned work'
'sad ... ?'
'stress ... ?'

The majority of what has been discussed and recommended so far represents the skills you need to develop first and foremost: those of respect (values), listening (behaviours) and placing patients first (attitudes). These principles and skills sets form the foundation of the consultation and the remainder of the consultation needs structuring logically and efficiently in order to meet the patient's agenda and your own agenda, as a doctor. A model of consultation can help you do this. While models are not intended to direct you robotically through every aspect from beginning to end they provide an excellent framework to develop good habits.

Choose a set of questions/phrases (as detailed in the tables in this chapter) for each stage of the consultation that you are comfortable using and memorise them. Remember the old adage, 'practice makes perfect'? Practice improves performance to varying degrees in all individuals but eventually renders most practised processes unconscious and habitual. Once you have developed a repertoire you will be more able to concentrate on what the patient is saying. Primarily, the successful exchange of information is the goal and the key to this is developing an effective strategy.

What's the evidence? Models of consultation

The latter quarter of the last century saw the emergence of a number of helpful models of consultation, with theoretical underpinnings constructed in the main from the disciplines of psychology, anthropology and sociology. Medical authors and, more latterly, nursing authors have adapted and integrated the ideology and applied these to the principles and constructs from their own disciplinary perspectives. Therefore, some are task- and skill-oriented, some process- and outcome-based, many focus on the relationship between clinician and patient and others aim to focus on patients' perspective of illness and are patient-centred; all are evolutionary (see 'Going Further' at the end of this chapter).

Figure 1.1 is a diagrammatic example of the synthesis of some of the models and shows how a framework can be developed to meet the needs of both clinician and patient. The enhanced Calgary–Cambridge approach (Kurtz et al., 2003) is the most commonly taught model in medical schools in the UK (18 out of 30 medical schools: Gillard et al., 2009). This approach is suitable for both primary care and secondary care settings. Please access the guide on the websites below, as it is extremely useful: www.skillscascade.com or http://www.gp-training.net/training/communication_skills/calgary/guide.htm.

You will find that the guides identify over 70 core, evidence-based communication process skills that fit into a framework of tasks and objectives. Addressing the inherent imbalance of power in the consultation aids the flow of information exchange and therefore increases the potential to move towards a shared plan of treatment which may or may not (but more likely will) include pharmacological intervention (Birks and Watt, 2007). Shared plans of treatment result in greater adherence by the patient to plans made and particularly to drug treatment regimes. An important adjunct for consideration here is the health economics element and the fact that non-adherence to medicines is enormously expensive. According to NICE (2009), the cost of unused or unwanted medicines in the NHS is estimated to be around £100 million annually.

Understanding, clarifying and making sense of the patient's perspective

The final element of the screening phase of the consultation is summarising back to the patient what you think the patient has described. If you haven't got it right or missed anything, the patient will (or should) correct you. Table 1.3 details a number of useful phrases to help you with final screening.

Table 1.3 Phrases for summarising and clarifying

'Before I examine you I just need to check that I've fully understood what you've told me today: you have … , have I got that right?'
'Now just so I know I have got to grips with all that's going on, you tell me that … : have I missed anything?'
'So just to make sure I've got things right, you have … , is that right?'
'Just to recap, you have had … anything else?'
'So I'll just summarise what you have told me … did I miss anything?'
'Can I just make sure I understand what you are telling me … is that correct?'

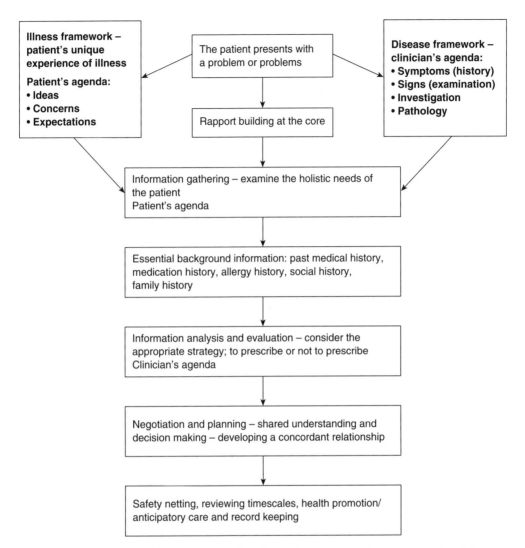

Figure 1.1   Patient-centred consultation, using the work of Berlin and Carter (2007) and the seven principles of good prescribing (NPC, 2007)

The next stage is exploration of the patients' ideas, concerns and expectations (ICE). Cues inform you what is important to the patient and needs responding to; in fact, noting and responding to these overt expressions of concern can be pivotal to the success of the consultation. Not all patients' cues are obvious – some are more subtle and therefore require a greater listening acuity.

The major pitfall here, in addition to missing cues at this stage in your consultation, is that unfortunately not all patients express what they are really thinking and feeling. Care needs to be taken now more than in any other area of soliciting information; if your ICE enquiry is not framed correctly it may be perceived as incompetence. For example, if you ask, 'So what is it you think you may have?' the patient will likely respond with 'I don't know, doctor, that's why I am here'. Patients may also take umbrage with phrases such as, 'What is it that

Table 1.4 Exploring patients' ideas, concerns and expectations (ICE)

'I have some ideas about what might be going on here but I just wanted to check if you have any thoughts about what it might be?'

'Have you considered what might be causing these problems?'

'Have you any thoughts as to what might be going on?'

'Many patients have concerns. I wonder if you have any?'

'You've mentioned a few things there; is there one you are particularly concerned about?'

'So from all of this is there anything specific that is worrying you?'

'When you said 'serious', what was going through your mind when you said that?'

'Is there anything particular or specific that you are uneasy about?'

'There are a couple of options to help you with this; it would be helpful if you could tell me what you were hoping I might do.'

'Had you any thoughts as to what we might be able to do for this?'

'You've obviously given this some thought; what were you thinking might be the best way of tackling this?'

you are worried about?' as this may imply additional meaning such as ill-founded anxiety on the part of the patient.

Table 1.4 details a number of useful phrases to help you when exploring ICE with patients.

Essential background medication information gathering

A thorough drug history is necessary to establish what medication the patient is taking, both prescribed and bought at a pharmacy and over the counter (OTC) at supermarkets and local stores. In some cases, drugs may be obtained from friends and relatives. You need to know this for a number of reasons, not least because it may be that the medication the patient is taking is the cause of the patient's presenting problem(s) or there may be contributing side-effects.

In Chapter 8 you will see that an important consideration is always to include the possibility of an adverse drug reaction in your differential diagnosis. It might be that the patient has had the presenting problem diagnosed previously and is not taking a prescribed drug treatment correctly or perhaps has not taken it at all. Enquiring whether the patient is taking prescribed medication as intended by the prescriber links well into determining whether the patient understands why the medication was prescribed in the first place and therefore whether the medication is still necessary.

Current medication may preclude the use of other medications due to a potential interaction between the two (see Chapter 9).

If you are clerking a patient for an inpatient stay in hospital, clearly the patient's regular medications will need to continue. Whether the patient is sensitive or allergic to any medication is crucial so that you do not inadvertently prescribe that treatment. In patients who give a history of allergy to a drug, establishing the history of the allergy and trying to ascertain whether the patient has a 'true' allergy is necessary as your first-line treatment options are narrowed if there are drugs that you cannot prescribe due to allergy (see Chapter 8). The patient's past medical history is important with reference to medication history as often patients can forget the drugs they take but will remember their medical conditions and, if prompted, can link them to a medication.

ACTIVITY 1.3 TAKING A MEDICATION HISTORY

List what you think constitutes a good medication history.

- What is a drug?
- What is medication?
- Is there a difference?
- In your general history taking, how would you enquire about illicit drugs?

Discuss your responses with colleagues to see if there are additional points for consideration.

What makes a good medication history?

You will hopefully have listed prescription-only medicines (POMs), pharmacy medicines (P) and OTC medications. More difficult here is the medications that patients do not always think of as 'drug medications'. Some patients think, for example, that herbal remedies are not important but in fact they have active ingredients that can interact with prescribed treatments or can be the cause of the patient's presenting problem (see Chapter 9).

Also treatments that have an alternative route other than by mouth (such as a suppository or an inhaler) can be perceived by the patient as not a drug medication. Therefore it is necessary to ask about specific 'remedies' or treatments that patients may have been prescribed but do not understand as medication and also those which they may be using to 'self-medicate'.

Table 1.5 details the mnemonic PAKASPO CHIPES that we have created to help you take a thorough medication history. You may feel that mnemonics should be simple words that you can remember. However, we have used this one for the past ten years with non-medical prescribers and have found it very successful. Taking time to learn it will reap rewards. Some mnemonics are so simple that users become confused about what they represent; this is not the case with this one.

This mnemonic does not take account of recreational drugs, smoking or alcohol. Using the mnemonic will help you to collect and harvest everything you need to ensure safety when moving on to deliberate and share with the patient your likely diagnosis and management. Look at the headings and think about how you might frame your enquiry about the patient's POMs and what you need to know other than the names of the drugs. Now think about how you will ask about patients' adherence to, and their knowledge of, the POMs they are taking.

Table 1.5 A mnemonic for efficient and effective medication history taking: PAKASPO CHIPES

- Prescription-only medicines
- Adherence
- Knowledge
- Allergies
- Side-effects
- Pharmacy-only medicines
- Over-the-counter medicines
- Creams, lotions, gels
- Herbal
- Inhalers
- Patches
- Eye/ear/nasal drops
- Suppositories/pessaries

The PAKASPO CHIPES framework involves some straightforward self-explanatory questioning (e.g. 'Do you use any creams, lotions or gels?') and some areas which require further expansion. It is not sufficient only to discover the name of the drugs the patient is taking: the dosage and frequency are also required in order to identify possible underdosage or overdosage and other non-therapeutic regimes.

Care also needs to be taken to avoid premature closure of medication questioning after the patient has listed two or three medications. This may occur when patients are taking several medications; they can lose track of what they have told you so far and stop. If you do not check and ask 'Anything else?' or 'Is that all your prescribed medicines?' you risk missing important drug information. If a patient is discharged from hospital having been started on a new drug or receives a prescription for a new drug at the surgery and has not had the treatment rationale explained, then it is understandable that the patient is less likely to take the recommended treatment. If patients do not know the purpose of their medication it is fairly hard to disguise this, and it is essential to tread carefully in order not to embarrass them.

ACTIVITY 1.4 WHY MIGHT PATIENTS NOT TAKE PRESCRIBED MEDICATION?

What do you understand about the term compliance?

The following phrases can be used to elicit the patient's adherence to prescribed medication. Identify which ones will keep the spirit of the consultation patient-centred and which have the power base firmly with the clinician:

- 'What medications are you supposed to be taking, but aren't?'
- 'What medications are you taking differently from the way you were told to take them?'

- 'Some people taking prescribed medicines stop taking them for a number of reasons; has that been the case for you?'
- 'I imagine that taking medication every day can be a hassle; do you ever have problems sticking to the treatment?'
- 'What medications are you taking in a way that is different from how you were asked to take them?'
- 'Some patients may stop taking medications when they shouldn't; is that the same for you?'
- 'These medications are quite important; you don't forget to take them, do you?'
- 'You are taking quite a few medications; it must be difficult to remember to take them; do you sometimes forget?'
- 'Do you sometimes stop taking your medication because you feel better, or in fact because you feel worse?'

Activity 1.4 challenged you to consider the word 'compliance' and think about the potential power connotations associated with the words you may use and how verbal and non-verbal interaction with patients may influence how you are ultimately perceived by patients. This is inextricably linked to why patients do or do not take prescribed treatments, although it is not simply about you as clinician; non-adherence is multifactorial and is a regularly researched issue. As we discussed earlier, it is expensive in terms of both human cost (poor health outcomes for patients) and in economic terms. The issues involved and how you might contribute to reducing both these costs are discussed later in this chapter.

Information analysis and evaluation

Following information gathering, your diagnostic reasoning ability and skills come into play. The judgements you make are influenced by your clinical knowledge and experience. You will now have a large amount of information that requires sifting and sorting in order to distinguish between the relevant and the irrelevant and, most importantly, exclude the dangerous. Always remember psychological and social factors influence health as well as the physiological, anatomical and biochemical (Gask and Usherwood, 2002). Having factored these elements into your reasoning and undertaken any necessary physical examination, what would you do next?

You may need to order tests or other investigations if there is still doubt as to the diagnosis. It is not always possible to come to a definitive diagnosis, therefore the main objective is to exclude the serious.

It is important and useful to find out what patients prefer in terms of the information you give. They may have had their condition for years and have become the 'lay expert'. Table 1.6 gives you some useful phrases to find out what the patient wants in terms of information.

Table 1.6 Phrases for establishing patients' preference and readiness for information

'I don't know how much you know about diabetes. It would be good if you could tell me what you already know so that I can fill in the gaps either now or later, whichever you prefer.'
'There's quite a lot of information on Parkinson's disease and the drugs used to treat it. Some people like as much information as possible immediately and others just want the bare essentials to start with. How much information would you like today?'
'I would like to discuss with you important information about asthma and the medication that can help. Some patients like to know a lot about these things and some wish to keep it to a minimum; how much information would you like?'

Negotiation and planning: shared understanding and decision making

In a frank and open environment you can discuss the options for treatment with the aim that you help the patient – the therapeutic objective of the consultation. Not all patients have a life-changing or an enduring problem that requires intervention and to do nothing might be the most beneficial therapeutic option. Watchful waiting, self-help strategies and perhaps OTC remedies can often be the most appropriate way forward. If the patient chooses a watchful waiting approach you should emphasise that you suspect the condition will settle over time but if additional signs and symptoms emerge your original diagnosis may need revising. Failure to communicate this can result in the patient thinking you have made an incorrect diagnosis.

If doing nothing is not an option and prescribing a drug treatment is the most appropriate therapeutic choice, then you need to consider the clinical purpose of prescribing. This is sixfold:

1. curative;

2. symptomatic relief;

3. disease-modifying;

4. empirical;

5. tactical;

6. preventive/prophylactic.

ACTIVITY 1.5 EXPLORING THE CLINICAL PURPOSES OF PRESCRIBING

Think about the six areas above and which drugs might achieve these clinical purposes. Two examples are given below: list one more example for each and then consider how you might explain the clinical purpose of the medication you are about to prescribe.

Curative example

Malathion lotion for scabies

Topical antibiotic drops for infective conjunctivitis

Symptomatic relief example

Non-steroidal anti-inflammatory drug such as ibuprofen for joint pain

Proton pump inhibitor such as lansoprazole for dyspepsia

Disease-modifying example

Methotrexate for rheumatoid arthritis

Beta-interferon and glatiramer acetate for multiple sclerosis

Empirical example

Antibiotics when symptoms are highly suggestive of a diagnosis – urgency and frequency on micturition probably indicate a urinary tract infection

Increasing sputum production and shortness of breath in a patient with chronic obstructive pulmonary disease is likely an exacerbation and requires antibiotic and oral steroid treatment

Tactical example

To gain time when collecting information such as a trial of β_2-agonist in a child with persistent nocturnal cough

A trial of a proton pump inhibitor in an adult with persistent cough

Preventive (prophylaxis) example

Inhaled corticosteroid in a patient with asthma

A statin in diabetic patients with normal cholesterol

(Fraser, 1999)

Once the therapeutic purpose of prescribing is clear to you then selecting a suitable (evidence-based) drug that meets the patient's profile (diagnosis, current and past medication, previous adverse drug reactions/allergy and past medical history) is usually straightforward. In the hospital setting you will be expected to prescribe within the formulary set by the Medicines Committee/Drug and Therapeutics Committees (see Chapter 3). In general practice there should be a practice formulary for you to refer to; however, take care, as evidence is changing at a rapid rate and you need a reliable regularly updated source, such as www.patient.co.uk, to refer to. This is a peer-reviewed online resource for both health professionals and patients and you can direct patients to this site or print off the patient information leaflet regarding both their condition and treatment. Having selected the most suitable first-line evidence-based drug for the patient, information about the drug should be provided in digestible portions with regular clarification of understanding, often referred to as 'chunking and checking' (UKCCC, 2006).

Conveying that medication is often only one part of the solution is important. Starting with small chunking of information and checking frequently for understanding helps you gauge the size of chunking needed later; how much information a patient wants or can take in varies and changes over time. However, there are a number of things that should always be explained at the time of the first prescription.

Having conveyed that there is not always a cure or 'quick fix', you also need to discuss the possibility that the first-line drug treatment chosen may not be the right one. Advice giving should include:

1. the dosage and frequency regime;

2. the duration of treatment;

3. possible side effects.

There are a number of techniques which will aid you in explaining medical aims, discussing the advantages and disadvantages of the proposed medicines, and checking understanding. The main objective is to help patients to recall information accurately later when deliberating on what has happened and make decisions which are based on correct information and their subjective and lived experiences. Patient recall is enhanced and increased by signposting, explicit categorisation, repetition and the use of diagrams (NICE, 2009). The information-gathering methods of summarisation and clarification/screening are continued throughout this phase also.

Give practical advice that can be followed and discuss how a structure can help by pinning the taking of medication with specific points in the day: 'Take this four times a day, before breakfast, lunch, evening meal and before bed', not 'Take this four times per day'. Be specific about important information: 'Take this with a full glass of water', not 'Take plenty of water'. Patients tend to remember instructions if they know why – 'Take this with food as it can cause stomach pain if you take it on an empty stomach', not 'Don't take this on an empty stomach'. Use patient information leaflets as you talk through the plans with the patient and highlight or underline important parts as you progress through each category (Table 1.7).

Defining compliance, adherence and concordance – word power

The majority of what has been discussed and recommended in the latter part of this chapter is leading you towards a concordant relationship.

Earlier you were asked what you understood by non-compliance. You may have understood the word to be benign and simply used when a patient has not complied with treatment instructions. It is particularly associated with medicine taking, although you may find it used to describe any patient non-adherence to instructions given to patients by clinicians. Compliance is defined as: *the extent to which the patient's behaviour matches the prescriber's recommendations* (Haynes *et al.*, 1979). Despite the simplicity of the definition, it has been criticised for having power

Table 1.7 Developing targeted information giving

The following phrases can be used to enhance patient recall and achieve a shared understanding:

Signposting

- 'I need to explain something very important'.
- 'I have a number of essential things you need to take away today'.

Repetition/summarising

- 'So, just to recap we have agreed to ... and you are going to take ... : does that sound about right?'
- 'We've covered a lot of ground here; I'll just summarise what we have agreed to do today'.

Checking understanding

- 'How do you feel now that I've explained that to you? What questions does it leave you with? Is there anything you would like me to go over again?'
- 'We have discussed a lot today and I'm worried that I might not have made it very clear. Could you tell me what we have agreed today so I can check I have explained it OK?'

---

connotations, with the power biased towards the clinician – 'do as I say' – and the patient being expected to follow 'the doctor's orders' passively.

The term adherence was adopted as a less demeaning alternative word to compliance in an attempt to emphasise that patients are free to decide whether to follow the prescriber's recommendations (Barofsky, 1978). Adherence develops the definition of compliance and is elevated slightly by emphasising the need for agreement. There is only one subtle change: *The extent to which the patient's behaviour matches the agreed recommendations of the prescriber.*

Marinker defines concordance as being:

> *based on the notion that the work of the prescriber and patient in the consultation is a negotiation between equals and that the aim is a therapeutic alliance between them. This alliance may include an agreement to differ. Its strength lies in an assumption of respect for the patient's agenda and the creation of openness in the relationship, so that both doctor and patient together can proceed on the basis of reality and not of misunderstanding, distrust or concealment.*

(Marinker, 1997, p. 8)

The Medicines Partnership (cited in Horne *et al.*, 2005) further developed this as an *alliance in which the health care professionals recognise the primacy of the patient's decisions about taking the recommended medications.*

Within the concept of non-compliance and non-adherence, the patient alone may be deemed responsible. However, concordance places the responsibility with the prescriber and the patient; there are two parties involved. The patient alone cannot be non-concordant; concordance is not another word for compliance. The terms compliance and non-compliance continue to be used every day in clinical practice and in the medical, nursing and pharmaceutical literature. Why do you think this might be?

Reviewing timescales, anticipatory care and record keeping

The final part of the consultation involves pulling together the negotiation, ensuring mutual understanding, checking for patient satisfaction regarding the plan, undertaking housekeeping and closing the encounter. Anticipatory care is the health promotion and disease prevention element and involves enhancing patients' responsibility for their own health. It may occur in a vacuum at the end of the consultation but often several opportunities present throughout the consultation.

Safety netting and reviewing timescales entail reiterating what needs to happen if the diagnosis is not correct or the treatment is not efficacious. In general practice, emergency departments and out-of-hours/walk-in centre settings, ruling out serious illness often takes priority over ruling in a specific diagnosis. Therefore safety netting and reviewing timescales are paramount and flow seamlessly from the information-giving stage of chunking and checking. Think about three phrases you could use to ensure that patients are aware of what to do if there is deterioration, side-effects or no change in their condition. Advising on timescales will depend upon the condition and the treatment. Revisit Activity 1.5, but this time think about the timescales and when you would expect the patient to notice benefit from treatment in each scenario and what you would recommend to the patient in each case.

Clarifying timescales naturally closes the consultation. Review the patient's knowledge, understanding and concerns about medicines at regular intervals agreed with the patient. Offer repeat information on every review, especially when treating patients with enduring long-term conditions and those taking multiple medicines.

Record keeping is the final task of the consultation for the clinician. Careful documentation not only helps you to remember why the decisions were made and the reasons certain actions were taken but also makes it clear to other clinicians who may be caring for the patient. Inadequate records can adversely affect patients and other colleagues; think about why. It is fair to say that the diagnostic process is complex and the demands of everyday practice are immense, and record keeping can be relegated and considered a less important part of the consultation. From a medicolegal point of view this adage says it all: 'If it isn't written down, it didn't happen.'

Conclusion

The consultation can be defined as a meeting between two experts:

- The doctor is expert in medicine (underlying pathology, differential diagnosis).
- The patient is expert in his or her illness (unique illness experience).
- Achieving a shared understanding is the aim.

(Tuckett *et al.*, 1985)

If you approach every patient encounter with these principles in mind, then patient-centred practice will become second nature to you, patients will be more likely to take their medicines safely and the likelihood of positive patient outcomes will increase. Ultimately there is improved satisfaction for both patients and clinicians.

Chapter summary

This chapter has described different models of consultation and has explained how using bio-psycho-social models which take account of cultural and existential dimensions can positively influence medicine-taking behaviours. In particular it introduced and defined the concepts of compliance, adherence and concordance. It developed the theme of patient-centred practice and the need to consider the attitudes, knowledge and communication skills involved. The overarching theme of the chapter was how to recognise how the application of these skills can help patients take medicines safely.

GOING FURTHER

Balint M (1958) *The Doctor, the Patient and His Illness.* London: Tavistock.

Coulter A and Ellins J (2007) Effectiveness of strategies for informing, education and involving patients. *British Medical Journal*, 335: 24–27.

Department of Health (2008) *High Quality Care for All – NHS Next Stage Review: Final Report.* London: Department of Health.

Dowell J, Jones A and Snadden D (2002) Exploring medication use to seek concordance with 'non-adherent' patients: A qualitative study. *British Journal of General Practice*, 52: 24–32.

Eisenberg L (1977) Disease and illness: Distinctions between professional and popular ideas of sickness. *Culture, Medicine and Psychiatry*, 1 (1): 9–23.

General Medical Council (2004) *Confidentiality: Protecting and providing information.* Available online at: www.gmc-uk.org/guidance

General Medical Council (2006) *Good Medical Practice.* Available online at: www.gmc-uk.org/guidance

General Medical Council (2008) *Consent: Patients and doctors making decisions together.* Available online at: www.gmc-uk.org/guidance

Horne R (2001) Compliance, adherence and concordance. In: Taylor K and Harding G (eds) *Pharmacy Practice Education.* London: Taylor & Francis.

Lewin S, Skea Z, Entwistle V, Zwarenstein M and Dick J (2007) Interventions for providers to promote a patient-centred approach in clinical consultations. *Cochrane Review.* The Cochrane Database of Systematic Reviews, 2.

Ley P (1988) *Communication with Patients: Improving satisfaction and compliance.* London: Croom Helm.

National Prescribing Centre. (2008) *Five Minute Guide: Quality prescribing.* Available online at: http://www.npc.nhs.uk/improving_safety/improving_quality/resources/5mg_qualityprescibing.pdf (accessed 9 July 2013).

Royal Free & University College Medical School. Available online at: www.faculty.
londondeanery.ac.uk (accessed 6 August 2012).

Shaller D (2007) *Patient Centred Care: What does it take?* Oxford: Picker Institute
and The Commonwealth Fund.

Thistlethwaite J, Evans R, Tie R and Heal C (2006) Shared decision making and
decision aids: A literature review. *Australian Family Physician*, 35 (7): 537–540.

World Health Organization (2003) *Adherence to Long-Term Therapies: Evidence for
action.* Geneva: World Health Organization.

chapter 2

Law, Ethics and Professional Responsibilities in Prescribing Practice

Monica Murphy and Catherine Gill

Achieving your medical degree

This chapter will help you begin to meet the following outcomes of *Tomorrow's Doctors* (General Medical Council (GMC), 2009):

17. (c) Safe and legal prescribing.

    (e) Disclosure of information on medicines.

19. (a) Record keeping.

23. (c) Understand roles and relationships between agencies and services.

It will also link to:

Good Medical Practice (GMC, 2013a)

and

Good Practice in Prescribing and Managing Medicines and Devices (GMC, 2013b), particularly paragraphs 21–29 and 67–73.

and

A Single Competency Framework for all Prescribers (National Prescribing Centre, 2012) 1:7, 1:10, 2:24, 3:25–37, 4:42, 4:45, 4:47, 5:48–52, 6:55, 7:61–62, 9:70 and 9:71.

Chapter overview

This chapter provides a brief outline to essential medicines-related legislation and the professional role you have as a doctor when prescribing medicinal products for the patients in your care. Prescribing appropriately, safely and responsibly is both a professional and public expectation. This chapter explores issues of accountability for your prescribing practice and how harm might arise with patients through negligent disclosure of information in relation to drugs and failures in prescribing processes.

After reading this chapter you will be able to:

- apply the essential legal and professional requirements for safe and accountable pre-scribing practice;
- describe key legislation relevant to medicines licensing and prescribing;
- develop an ethical appreciation of the demands of prescribing;
- discuss consent in the context of information disclosure in prescribing practice;
- identify the potential for conflict of interests in your prescribing practice;
- recognise reliable sources of further information concerning safe and legal prescribing practice.

Introduction

Prescribing for patients is an essential and commonplace activity for doctors. It is difficult to imagine many clinical management situations where prescribing is not a feature. Safe prescribing, like every other area of practice, requires you to be informed so you can work in the patient's best interests. You should not be subject to coercion and you must be able to account for your decisions and actions.

Over time, legislation has been introduced that regulates the licensing, supply and sale of medicinal products. Such legislation sits alongside your ethical and legal obligations related to information disclosure, negotiating treatment outcomes and obtaining valid consent.

ACTIVITY 2.1 WHAT CONSTITUTES A LEGAL PRESCRIPTION?

Make a list of what information you think is necessary for a safe and legal prescription. You may wish to discuss this with a senior colleague and see if you both agree.

Now read the *Prescription Writing* section of the most recent copy of the *British National Formulary* (BNF). How does this compare to your list?

Your response should be written in ink, indelible print or secure approved electronic transmission. It should include:

- prescriber's name, profession, signature and reference number;
- patient's full name and address, age if under 12. Inclusion of date of birth is good practice;
- for each medicinal product – name, quantity, pharmacological form and strength;
- appropriate date – date of signing. (A repeatable prescription is one where more than one direction to dispense is indicated: see Chapter 1.) It requires the number of times for dispensing but if this is not specified then no more than two issues within 6 months from the date the prescription was signed. For further information, see the National Prescribing Centre guidelines on repeatable dispensing (National Prescribing Centre, 2008).

Clinical management should be regarded as a partnership between you the prescriber and the patient in your care. When you issue a prescription to a patient it is as a consequence of, and in response to, the clinical criteria the patient presents.

Concordance (see Chapter 1) is more likely to be achieved when patients fully understand the function and role medicines play in their clinical management. This requires them to have information on the drug, including what it's for, the route of administration, dose, precautions or special instructions and known common side-effects. Identified risks associated with the medicine plus the information you give should be recorded when the patient consents to the treatment.

Legislation and medicines

The 1968 Medicines Act legislates for the licensing of all medicinal products that claim to have a relevant medicinal action or function. A medicinal product is therefore understood as any administered substance that is used in the diagnostic processes or in the treatment and prevention of disease. In the UK, the Medicines Act encompasses all processes involved in the manufacture, marketing, advertisement, wholesale and supply of medicinal products.

Currently the BNF has around 6,000 medicines within it, many of which are potent and require very careful monitoring. The increase in the number and potency of medicines since the establishment of the NHS is one reason for the Act. Another is the thalidomide tragedy. There was little in the way of robust quality assurance, safety monitoring or scrutinising the effectiveness of products claiming to have a medicinal usage prior to the 1968 Medicines Act, although most historical legislation prior to this aimed to deal with poisons or known harmful substances. The Medicines Act also covers the labelling of medicinal products and the criteria for the containers used.

The purpose of the Human Medicines Regulations in 2012 (fully implemented by 2015) is to synthesise the key aspects of the Medicines Act 1968 with the many subsequent medicines regulations. It also dovetails and brings the UK in agreement with relevant European legislation and guidelines (see the European Medicines Agency: http://www.ema.europa.eu/ema). The overarching aim of the Human Medicines regulations is to reduce the risk and harm to patients from drugs and improve and provide consistency in managing drug safety, thereby assuring public health through transparent reporting processes.

Medicinal product licensing

The Medicines and Healthcare Products Regulatory Agency (MHRA: see www. mhra.gov.uk/index.htm) was founded as a result of the enactment of the Medicines Act. The MHRA is responsible for licensing medicinal products and quality assuring safety issues such as clinical trials and the clinical effectiveness of products. The MHRA is independent from the pharmaceutical industry. Of necessity, the approval and licensing processes of a medicinal product are robust and subject to strict testing. For further information on the process, see www.mhra.gov.uk/Howweregulate/Medicines/Licensingofmedicines/index.htm.

Once a licence (marketing authorisation – MA) previously known as a product licence, and which you still see on medicine packs, is issued by the MHRA, it usually lasts for 5 years. The MHRA continues to monitor medicinal products by collating the information supplied by the Yellow Card Scheme for suspected adverse drug reactions and has the authority to revoke an MA (see Chapter 8).

The Medicines Act classifies medicinal products as:

- prescription-only medicines (POM);
- general sales list (GSL);
- pharmacy medicines (P).

POMs, as you might expect, require a valid prescription from an appropriate practitioner in order for them to be supplied or sold. Most POMs can be supplied under Patient Group Directions (see Chapter 4).

GSL medicines can be purchased from non-pharmacy premises (e.g. supermarkets, garage forecourt shops). GSL medicines are sold in the manufacturer's packs and the dose, strength and pack size are restricted. As its name implies, this is a list of named preparations and this list can be amended as necessary. If it was thought that a GSL preparation was being abused, then it could be reclassified as P or even POM.

P medicines are those which can be supplied without a prescription but under the supervision and personal control of a pharmacist in suitably registered premises. Drugs can also be deregulated from POM to P or from P to GSL. Two examples of changes from POM to P are omeprazole and diclofenac, though the P packs may be in lower doses, restricted age groups or smaller pack sizes than the POM equivalent. In the case of naproxen, for example, it can be sold to the public for the treatment of dysmenorrhoea in women aged between 15 and 50 years subject to a maximum single dose of 500mg and a maximum daily dose of 750mg for a maximum of 3 days. There is also a restriction on the pack size that can be sold. A drug which moved from POM to P and then to GSL is ranitidine. This can be sold as a GSL, again with age restrictions (adults only) and for a maximum pack size. The strength is also restricted to 75mg as a single dose and a maximum daily dose of 300mg.

Less frequently, medicines which were previously classified as P are made POM if new risks are identified which require involvement of a doctor to ensure safe use of the medicine. In the same way a GSL medicine could be reclassified as P if new information showed that it was no longer safe to supply it without a pharmacist checking that it was suitable for the patient.

(MHRA, 2012, reclassification criteria)

Misuse of drugs

Any drug can be misused, but this is particularly true for drugs that can lead to dependency and addiction. The 1971 Misuse of Drugs Act and subsequent regulations legislate for the limits and controls placed on those drugs which by their very nature can pose risk in relation to addiction, altered psychological states or an ability to enhance performance (e.g. some sporting activities) or cause hallucinogenic effects. The intention of placing certain prohibitions and restrictions on these drugs is to minimise their misuse or inappropriate use.

The drugs encompassed by this legislation are therefore controlled – the control element relating to the possession, supply, sale and use of the drug. The Misuse of Drugs Act covers not only licensed medicinal products but also those drugs that have a non-medicinal use. Regulations subsequent to this Act, e.g. the Misuse of Drugs Regulations 2001, set out the classification and medicinal schedules for drugs.

Scenario 2.1: Too many prescription requests

Mr Taylor puts in a prescription request via the reception at your group practice surgery for codeine 30mg, 1 to 2 four times daily, 100 tablets, stating that he lost the last prescription issued to him. You note from his record that in the last 8 months this is the third time Mr Jones has asked for this drug early and each time it has been issued from a different prescriber in your practice. You suspect that Mr Jones may be misusing or even selling on his prescribed medication.

What issues does this scenario raise for you? What are the possible actions you could take and how would you justify them?

Efficient prescription recording systems within practice should alert you to earlier than usual requests for a repeat prescription, even if the patient approaches several prescribers. This scenario also demonstrates that continuity of care and accurate prescribing records are essential to the identification of potential abuse.

Doing nothing is not an option. You need to:

- discuss your concerns with Mr Taylor openly;
- listen sympathetically and decide if a change in his condition is the reason for the potential increase in use;
- involve a senior colleague to help resolve the issue;
- involve the practice manager and other prescribers in the practice to ensure the system is being used effectively.

The Misuse of Drugs Regulations 2001

These authorise the legitimate use of controlled drugs (CDs) and who can legally prescribe, possess and supply them. The key areas that the regulations consider are:

- administering and dispensing CDs;
- record keeping (including the CD Register);
- safe storage of drugs;
- destruction of drugs and their disposal.

There are three classes of CD (A, B and C). The classification is for the purpose of establishing penalties under law, with the most severe penalties applied according to the higher the classification of drug, A being the highest.

Classification can change: in 2001 cannabis was reclassified from B to C – the lower class – following the findings of the Runciman Inquiry (Police Foundation, 1999), but this classification was reversed in 2008.

The 2001 regulations also divide CDs into five schedules. These schedules are based on the regulation of the drug's use and potential for harm when it is misused, the seriousness of the consequences from misuse and the drug's therapeutic value.

- Schedule 1 CDs are not for medical use and are subject to Home Office licence. They include drugs such as cannabis and LSD.

- Schedule 2–5 drugs are of concern to you as a prescriber. Possession of a schedule 2 drug without appropriate authority (e.g. a valid prescription) could be subject to prosecution.

It will be of benefit to you to discuss with a pharmacist colleague what drugs are contained within the various schedules. You could also find out what happens in your area of practice, where the CD cupboard is, who checks the contents, the location of the CD Register, and what happens when patients prescribed CDs move from one clinical area to another.

Prescribing controlled drugs

Since the revision of existing regulations (the Misuse of Drugs Regulations) and the introduction of others (The Controlled Drugs – Supervision of Management and Use Regulations 2006) along with adopting some of the recommendations of the Fourth Report of the Shipman Inquiry (2004), the prescribing of CDs has been subject to much tighter controls and monitoring than previously. It should be noted that you, as a doctor, may not use a patient-specific prescription in order to replenish practice stocks or your personal doctor's bag stock.

Except for the appropriate treatment of severe and acute pain you should not prescribe schedule 2 drugs to a known CD addict unless you possess a Home Office licence for treating addicts. In addition to the essential requirements for a valid prescription, you should follow the guidelines in your latest copy of the BNF concerning prescribing CDs.

Dispensing doctors

In remote and rural areas where patients live above a prescribed distance from a pharmacy, there is provision for doctors to dispense medicinal products from their surgery premises. Those who dispense need to be particularly vigilant in reducing the opportunity for error when they are also responsible for writing the prescription. For further information on dispensing doctors and the regulations that affect dispensing practice, visit http://www.dispensingdoctor.org.

Repeat prescribing

General practice is the place for repeat prescribing systems; in fact, repeat prescribing accounts for 60–70% of prescription costs and 80% of prescription items in primary care (Department of Health, 2007). Patients can usually request a repeat prescription over the phone or online.

However, in hospital, where repeat prescribing is rare, if you have seen a patient as an inpatient or in one of the clinics and have recommended a long-term treatment in a letter to the patient's GP, are you reassured that the patient will continue to receive the appropriate medications when discharged from your care?

There are some drugs where repeat prescribing may not be appropriate or may be limited, usually because they are particularly potent and monitoring is needed prior to a prescription being issued. Examples could be methotrexate, warfarin or lithium. In these cases you need to see the blood results prior to offering a prescription. Renal and hepatic dysfunction may result in a change of dose or drug.

With lithium you may offer a repeat prescription to those who are stable but limit the number of repeats to two or three before a patient review is required.

Evidence of monitoring must be available to you as the prescriber before a repeat prescription is issued. The duration of repeat prescriptions for other drugs such as disease-modifying antirheumatic drugs should be limited to ensure that prescriptions are actively reviewed. Responsibility to define the issue number lies with you.

Repeat dispensing

Firstly, what do you understand by the term repeat dispensing?

NHS prescriptions could not be repeated until April 2005 (PSNC and BMA, 2009), although the Department of Health guidance was published in 2002 (see the Going Further list at the end of this chapter for more details).

Repeat dispensing is defined as:

> an alternative model for prescribing and dispensing regular medicines to patients on stable long-term treatment, where repeat supplies are managed by the patient's pharmacy of choice.
>
> (PSNC and BMA, 2009, p. 4)

It allows the prescriber to offer an NHS prescription with a number of repeats for a period of up to 12 months. Unlike the single private repeat prescription, for the NHS, the prescriber issues the number of paper prescriptions related to the number of repeats required. Each script will have a note of which one it is, for example, 1 of 6, 2 of 6, etc. The patient can retain the unused prescriptions or they can be stored in the pharmacy for collection. You need to be conscious of the need to monitor patients regularly and provide repeats in line with this. The published guidance on repeat dispensing gives some examples of where it might be of particular relevance.

Examples are patients:

- on single, stable therapy, for example, levothyroxine;
- with stable long-term conditions on multiple therapy, for example, hypertension;
- with diabetes or asthma who can appropriately self-manage seasonal conditions such as hayfever.

You can probably think of other areas that might be suitable for repeat dispensing as long as patient safety is not compromised.

Consent in the prescribing context

Personal autonomy and the availability of choices can be understood as the two essential ingredients for a person to consent (or provide an informed consent) to treatment. Without being presented with treatment options the individual lacks the context for making a decision. Without the ability to be self-determining (autonomous) when faced with decisions to be made about treatment, individuals lack the necessary opportunity to consider what would be appropriate for them and what represents their values, beliefs and treatment goals.

It is not enough that individuals merely assent to a clinical management plan that is proposed to them; they should be invited to engage and be concordant with the management plan. This requires discussion and negotiation. As a minimum it requires that the patient receives sufficient information to make a decision.

Lack of capacity

Drug and other medically related information needs to be explained in terms that the individual can understand, believe to be relevant and true, retain and weigh up before acting upon. In the context of prescribing, the information you provide to your patient regarding drugs must be factual, outlining the therapeutic actions, risks, alternatives and benefits plus any unique or cautionary issues (e.g. side-effects or special instructions).

Under the Mental Capacity Act 2005 you must always assume a patient possesses the capability to make a decision unless it is established that he or she lacks capacity at the particular time when the decision needs to be made. Patients with limited, diminishing and fluctuating capacity may still be able to understand and retain sufficient information that is material to the decision to be made and thereby provide a valid consent to treatment. In the event that a patient does lack capacity, decisions concerning treatment are made in consideration of the existence of a valid advance directive and the patient's best interests.

Liability in prescribing

As the GMC (2012) report on prescribing in general practice demonstrated, errors with prescriptions are common but do not usually have severe consequences. Errors can occur in the prescribing itself, e.g. dose/route, in the monitoring of patients, e.g. suboptimal monitoring and/or not ordering tests, and are likely to increase in frequency the more drugs a patient is prescribed. Identified errors associated with the prescriber indicated that insufficient drug knowledge and perception of risk were factors. In some established doctors, their experience can induce a tendency towards complacency, particularly when prescribing for longer-term patients, and they may thereby overlook the relevant caveats applicable to effective clinical management. Areas for particular concern relating to prescription errors include:

- incorrect dose;
- incorrect route for administration;
- ambiguous/illegible writing;
- prescribing a known patient allergen;
- lack of diligence – prescribing and inducing a drug interaction.

When these prescribing issues are added to significant factors associated with patients' ability to understand their proposed clinical management (e.g. language difficulties, limited literacy skills), the need for accuracy both in writing the prescription and communicating essential aspects of the medicines regime to patients becomes clear.

See also Chapter 7 for errors in prescribing.

Standards for information disclosure

Consider how you give information to patients, parents and carers. What do you include and why? How do you decide on the priorities and the weight that you associate with the explanations given? Do you give patients additional materials such as leaflets as an adjunct to your information or as the principal source of information? How you give information concerning medications is as relevant as what information you give.

What counts as sufficient information is not always easy to establish. An objective standard for disclosure is known as the prudent-patient view – what a reasonable or responsible patient would want to know (Mason and Laurie, 2011). This reflects an application of Bolam (the standard of a reasonable and responsible body of medical opinion). The Bolam test holds that the law imposes a duty of care, but the standard of that care is a matter of medical judgement.

The prudent-practitioner view suggests a more subjective approach and includes what the prescriber ranks as important to disclose. With the advent of negligence-related legal cases that challenge the content and degree of disclosure (see Chapter 4 of Mason and Laurie, 2011 for a discussion of *Sidaway v Board of Governors of the Bethlem Royal Hospital*, 1984; *Chester v Afshar*, 2005) an acceptable standard probably lies somewhere between subjective and objective.

Whilst there may appear to be imprecision as to what constitutes sufficient information provided to inform a decision, this can in part be gauged by the dialogue you have with your patient. The greater the complexity, need for monitoring or potential for toxicity of the drug regimen, the more comprehensive your information should be.

This also is a reminder of the importance of questions that patients ask as these can help determine the degree of significance that patients attach to perceived risks, even if you, the prescriber, do not view the risks with the same importance. These are material to the decision that a patient makes. Often, the prescribing management options are unlikely to be of the take-it-or-leave-it type and here you must also use professional judgement in recounting the various merits of drug regimens available without overwhelming the patient with choices that might seem quite close in action or application.

Liability and claims for medical negligence related to non-disclosure of information in the consent process are a relatively recent occurrence and are more likely to succeed if the claimant can demonstrate that the standards and duty of care owed him or her regarding disclosure of information were breached and were shown to be the cause of harm inflicted. For any claim of medical negligence to be successful claimants must be able to establish the following three principles:

1. A duty of care was owed to them.

2. The standard attached to that duty was not met.

3. Harm was caused by that breach of duty.

In relation to prescribing this can refer to what you prescribe (act) and your failure to prescribe (omission). Whilst the vigilant dispensing pharmacist and/or other healthcare professionals who may subsequently administer the prescribed drugs can question and intervene where a prescription is incorrect, the first duty lies with the prescriber to avoid error.

Off-label medicinal products prescribing

ACTIVITY 2.2 PRESCRIBING DRUGS OUTSIDE OF THEIR PRODUCT LICENCE

What is your understanding about prescribing a licensed medication outside its product licence, often described as off-label prescribing?

What do you think you should consider before prescribing any product outside its product licence?

The MHRA controls the MA of medicinal products. An MA is required for the supply or sale of a medicinal product. This MA functions to quality assure the product and identifies the dose, route of administration, contraindications, necessary patient monitoring and how the drug is to be used – known as a Summary of Product Characteristics (SPC). Prescribing off-label and unlicensed medicinal products requires well-thought-out professional judgement that is based on reliable and robust evidence. An off-label drug is one that is licensed for a particular use/medical treatment/age group, but which is prescribed outside its licence, e.g. amitriptyline (antidepressant) prescribed for neurogenic pain. It is not uncommon to prescribe off-label but you must ensure that the drug is safe, has proven efficacy, particularly in relation to licensed alternatives, and is in the patient's best interests (GMC, 2013b).

Case Study 2.1: Off-label prescribing

Mr Singh was diagnosed with migraine a number of years ago. During the last 6 months he has been suffering up to four attacks a month and has been debilitated by this frequency. You discussed prophylactic treatment with him and initially prescribed pizotifen. The frequency of attacks has reduced but unfortunately he is drowsy all day.

You now propose prescribing sodium valproate. This would be an off-label use for this medication. What issues does prescribing this, or any, off-label medicinal product raise?

In order to elicit a valid consent to taking this drug as part of Mr Singh's clinical management and establish concordance, what information do you consider to be essential and optional to be given to him?

Take care to explain that the drug is off-label and what this means; this is particularly important as the patient information leaflet that comes with the dispensed drug could be confusing to the patient. Ensure you understand and maintain an appropriate standard of knowledge regarding the medicinal product and its usage.

Only prescribe within your area of competency and experience. This may mean only prescribing following transfer of patient care (e.g. consultant to GP) after initial prescribing from a consultant and/or senior medical colleague. Responsibility for monitoring and reviewing the patient whilst taking the drug usually lies with the consultant who commenced the drug treatment. However, remember that liability lies with the individual who signs the prescription.

First, explore with Mr Singh any possible precipitating trigger factors. See the *Prophylaxis of Migraine* section of the most recent copy of the BNF for the most common provoking factors. Discuss with Mr Singh all other reasonable treatment options, such as the acute management of his migraine. Can no other licensed drug meet the needs for Mr Singh's condition? Consider Mr Singh's personal circumstances, e.g. previous drug adherence, lifestyle and preferences.

Is this the best option for Mr Singh? See the options for prophylactic treatment of migraine in the BNF and you will see that there are a number of unlicensed options. There is however no information regarding which option may be more likely to be beneficial to Mr Singh.

According to the Scottish Intercollegiate Guidelines Network (2008), sodium valproate has a number needed to treat (NNT) of 3.2 for reducing migraine effect by 50% or more compared with placebo. Topiramate should be initiated by a specialist due to side-effects and has an NNT of 3.9. Gabapentin has an NNT of 3.3.

Be satisfied that Mr Singh has provided a valid consent to undertake the treatment regime, record this and the content of your discussion and create an alert for follow-up with Mr Singh.

Always check for allergies and if he has ever taken this drug before. Are there likely to be any adverse effects? Then explain the drug's action and common side-effects. Explain what the drug does. Explain how to take the drug and confirm a review date. Inform Mr Singh that he must return if he has any problems or difficulties with the drug.

Optional information: respond to Mr Singh's questions. If he does not have any, then ask if he requires further clarification. Ask him to repeat back key elements of the essential information that you have provided – how to take the drug, attending for follow-up.

Prescribing off-label presents a degree of risk to you because the MHRA has not considered the therapeutic use of the medicinal product in the context for which you are prescribing it. Liability (negligence) for medicinal product failure is most likely to lie with the manufacturer. But if a medicinal product is prescribed and used outside its product licence then liability for patient harm caused by that product shifts to the prescriber. This becomes all the more important with regard to prescribing an unlicensed drug – a drug that is not licensed for any use/medical treatment or age group.

Accountability in prescribing practice

As a doctor you are accountable for your prescribing activity in a variety of domains:

- to your patients through your impartial and informed clinical judgements;
- to your profession (via the GMC);
- to the legal system (NHS fraud, civil and criminal jurisdictions);
- to your employer (General Medical Services contract, the clinical governance frameworks and your employment contract).

Accountability can be questioned under one or more domains and you should make every effort to ensure your prescribing practice is safe, free from bias and in the patient's best interests.

Influences on prescribing practice

There can be a variety of influences on prescribing practice. You should expect over the length of your career to become familiar with many commonly prescribed drugs as well as newly developed and introduced drugs that improve on previous treatments and which provide new and effective treatments where choices were limited or absent. Keeping up to date and informed on prescribing issues is a clinical responsibility and duty.

Pharmaceutical company relations

The Bribery Act 2010 refers to advantages, defined as gifts, payments and hospitality, given as inducements or rewards in order to respond in a way that favours the gift giver. Ceding to inducements for commercial or personal advantage can be punishable by a fine or up to 10 years' imprisonment. It is not unusual for grateful patients to offer a gift of gratitude after treatment, and to refuse might give offence. The arbiter of your decision to accept an individual gift should be based on the reasonableness of the gift and its proportionality. For example, a bottle of wine or box of chocolates is different in scale to the gift of a new car or the use of a holiday home for 2 weeks.

There should also be consideration of context. A workplace lunch funded by a pharmaceutical company during a presentation of product information and research updates can be both proportionate and reasonable. One principle of the Bribery Act concerns monitoring and it is here that a degree of personal judgement as well as robust systems within your organisation, e.g. NHS Trust or GP practice, is important in relationships with pharmaceutical companies and their representatives.

This is a good opportunity to find out what your Trust policy is towards pharmaceutical company representatives and towards any gifts or inducements they may offer. Try to locate a copy of the guidelines and read them. Do you feel your colleagues generally adhere to these guidelines? The National Prescribing Centre, which is now a part of the National Institute for Health and Care Excellence (NICE), sets out the boundaries for appropriate pharmaceutical industry contact. You must never allow any inducement, favour, sponsorship or reward to influence your prescribing practice.

Just as you should not be influenced by inducements in your prescribing practice, you should also consider the potential for coercion. Consider the following scenario.

Scenario 2.2: Exploring prescribing decisions

Jenny presents at your surgery with her 12-week-old baby son. She has previously attended with him for immunisations and ceased breastfeeding when he was 2 weeks old. Jenny reports that following a recommendation from another mum at a local playgroup she has bought a soya-based infant formula from the pharmacy and has been feeding her baby with this. She reports that he is settled and happy on this formula. She requests you to pre-scribe this infant formula for her. What issues does this scenario raise for prescribing?

If there were no clinical reasons to prescribe the infant formula for Jenny's baby, what might be your actions and how would you justify them?

If there is no clinical indication why this infant formula should be prescribed, then there is no compelling reason to do so.

Consider the consequences of prescribing and not prescribing.

Prescribing establishes a precedent and, in this case, for repeat prescribing that may end up with Jenny and/or others that she informs coming back and asking for prescriptions for items that are not clinically justified or which can be obtained over the counter. A simple refusal to prescribe the formula without further probing whether Jenny has other concerns could damage the doctor–patient relationship.

Ask if she is coping. Jenny's request for the prescription may be her ticket of admission for the consultation but not necessarily the real reason why she is seeking help.

It is possible that limited personal finances have prompted her to seek prescribed food for her baby. Consider who you might refer her to and how you might feasibly offer continued support.

Prescribing for family, self and non-registered patients

With group general practices, walk-in centres and one-stop shops finding an appropriate prescriber means that most visitors can reasonably access treatment at short notice when they cannot consult their usual doctor.

Non-registered patients (e.g. homeless persons, overseas tourists, asylum seekers) can be refused medical treatment if the grounds to do so are reasonable but in an emergency you can provide appropriate care that includes prescribing. Treating any patient who is unknown to you can present potential problems related to obtaining a thorough medical/drug history and continuity of care. In the case of a visiting non-registered patient who may have run out of his or her usual medication there is the additional factor of ensuring the correct drug and dose.

Wherever possible and with the consent of the patient, communication with the usual medical practitioner should occur prior to prescribing and certainly after treatment (GMC, 2013b). Treating overseas visitors (including asylum seekers and those who have been refused stay, who should firstly be considered on a humanitarian basis) in the NHS is subject to complex and complicated chargeable services, although there are reciprocal arrangements with European Economic Area countries (Department of Health, 2010).

ACTIVITY 2.3 PRESCRIBING FOR FRIENDS AND FAMILY

Have you ever been placed in a position where a colleague or family member needed a prescription? What did or would you do? What if it was a good friend – or yourself? What ethical considerations are there to prescribe for these people?

Discuss your responses with colleagues and see if they agree. This is an important consideration as if it has not yet happened the likelihood is that it will.

From your discussion and reflecting further you should be able to justify all decisions to prescribe. You may consider some prescribing, for medical colleagues, as being pragmatic and expedient as doing so allows them not to have to take time off and also to treat relatively minor ailments. However, one could regard this as blasé and open to abuse. If what should be exceptional becomes commonplace then you should challenge that practice.

Prescribing for colleagues, friends or family members should be considered as rare and unavoidable. You run the risk of lacking objectivity in your decisions when dealing with close friends or family members. You might prescribe when you normally would have pursued further investigations, exceed the limits of your competency or create an expectation that is not defensible (GMC, 2013b).

The advisability of prescribing CDs, with good reason, is even more circumscribed (GMC, 2013b) and limited to the most exceptional situations. You should be able to justify, both professionally and ethically, your necessity to prescribe and, with the patient's consent, inform the relevant GP of the prescription you have provided. Prescribing for yourself is to be considered with equal gravity. It was a recommendation of the Shipman Inquiry Fourth Report (2004) that self-prescribing of CDs becomes a criminal offence. Again, self-prescribing should never be a matter of convenience, time saving or complacency but should only ever be justified from the perspective of necessity and immediacy.

Chapter summary

In this chapter you have been introduced to key legislation relating to the regulation and use of medicinal products, essential requirements for prescribing and obtaining informed consent for treatment that includes prescribed drugs. In the activities you have had the opportunity to explore clinical practice and the potential challenges that prescribing can present. These challenges include ethical practice relating to freedom from influence or coercion plus pragmatic issues such as treating colleagues and challenging suspected misuse of drugs. Prescribing is likely to be an everyday activity that you will undertake in your clinical work and it is important that you understand the legal parameters for safe and defensible practice.

GOING FURTHER

Department of Health (2002) *Repeat Prescribing Guidelines.* www.dh.gov.uk/en/Publicationsandstatistics/Publications/PublicationsPolicyAndGuidance/DH_4009188

Hibberd R, Barber N, Cornford T and Lichtner V (2012) *The Evaluation of the Electronic Prescription Service in Primary Care: Interim report on the findings from the evaluation in early implementer sites.* Available online at: http://www.ucl.ac.uk/pharmacy/documents/staff_docs/EPS

Medicines and Healthcare Products Regulatory Authority. Available online at: http://www.mhra.gov.uk/#page=DynamicListMedicines (accessed 4 December 2012).

National Patient Safety Agency. Available online at: http://www.nrls.npsa.nhs.uk (accessed 4 December 2012).

NICE Medicines and Prescribing Support. Available online at: http://www.nice.org.uk/mpc

The National Prescribing Centre was integrated into NICE in 2011 and now provides advice and support for delivering quality, safety and efficiency in the use of medicines.

Standard General Medical Services – Model contract and variation document (2010) Available online at: www.dh.gov.uk/en/Publicationsandstatistics/Publications/PublicationsPolicyAndGuidance/DH_116299 (accessed 4 December 2012).

The Human Medicines Regulations (2012) and The Medicines Act (1968): see respectively http://www.mhra.gov.uk/Howweregulate/Medicines/Overviewofmedicineslegislationandguidance/TheHumanMedicines Regulations2012/index.htm and http://www.legislation.gov.uk/ukpga/1968/67/contents

chapter 3

Evidence-based Practice and Keeping Up To Date

Andy Hutchinson and Jonathan Underhill

Achieving your medical degree

This chapter will help you begin to meet the following requirements of *Tomorrow's Doctors* (General Medical Council (GMC), 2009):

11. (f) Evaluate and apply epidemiological data in managing healthcare for the individual and the community.

12. Apply scientific method and approaches to medical research.

    (a) Critically appraise the results of relevant diagnostic, prognostic and treatment trials and other qualitative and quantitative studies as reported in the medical and scientific literature.

    (b) Formulate simple relevant research questions in biomedical science, psychosocial science or population science, and design appropriate studies or experiments to address the questions.

    (c) Apply findings from the literature to answer questions raised by specific clinical problems.

13. The graduate will be able to carry out a consultation with a patient:

    (f) Determine the extent to which patients want to be involved in decision-making about their care and treatment.

19. Use information effectively in a medical context.

    (d) Access information sources and use the information in relation to patient care, health promotion, giving advice and information to patients, and research and education.

    (e) Apply the principles, method and knowledge of health informatics to medical practice.

It will also link to:

Good Medical Practice (GMC, 2013a)

and

Good Practice in Prescribing and Managing Medicines and Devices (GMC, 2013b), particularly paragraphs 6–11.

Chapter overview

A large part of your job as a doctor is to make decisions. Evidence-based medicine (EBM) is founded on the idea that decision making in healthcare should incorporate the best available evidence in conjunction with the experience of the clinician and the views of the patient (Sackett *et al.*, 1996). Failure to use evidence in the best possible way leads to inefficiency and a reduction in both quality and quantity of life for patients. This chapter will help you keep up to date with current evidence, sift the good from the not so good evidence and manage information overload.

After reading this chapter you will be able to:

- describe how humans make decisions, using the language of dual-process theory, and reflect on the implications of this for your practice;
- distinguish between useful and less useful information by filtering for relevance and validity;
- apply principles of information mastery to keep up to date with the evidence base.

ACTIVITY 3.1

In the NHS, evidence-based guidance is sometimes under or over implemented, with considerable variations in uptake (NHS Information Centre, 2011).

Think about why this should be. What are the barriers to practising medicine in an evidence-based way? How could you address these? Think about this now, make a list and come back to it to see if you want to change or add anything after you have read the chapter.

What is evidence-based medicine?

Probably the most widely used definition of evidence-based medicine (EBM) is that provided by Sackett *et al.*:

> *Evidence-based medicine is the conscientious, explicit, and judicious use of current best evidence in making decisions about the care of individual patients. The practice of evidence-based medicine means integrating individual clinical expertise with the best available external clinical evidence from systematic research.*

> (Sackett *et al.*, 1996, p. 71)

It's important to note that, in this definition, *clinical expertise* includes the proficiency and judgement that individual practitioners like you acquire through experience, and the incorporation of patients' perspectives and preferences into decisions.

How far does this definition take us? Taken at face value it simply seems to say that EBM is the wise use of the best available evidence. Surely that is what health professionals have been doing for centuries. Would you like to be cared for by someone who expressly chooses not to take note of the best available evidence?

We need to think about what we mean by 'evidence'.

What do we mean by 'evidence'?

In the context of EBM, *best available external clinical evidence* means the evidence about how well a therapy works and what risks are associated with it that is most likely to be accurate and least likely to be incorrect. An alternative definition of EBM, first proposed by Greenhalgh and Donald in 2002, helps clarify what we mean by the 'E' in EBM:

> *The use of mathematical estimates of the chance of benefit and the risk of harm, derived from high-quality research on population samples, to inform clinical decision-making.*

> (Greenhalgh, 2012, p. 94)

Different hierarchies of evidence have been suggested, but they all rate objective experimental study designs, such as randomised controlled trials (RCTs), above observational studies, such as cohort and case-control studies; and these above expert opinion and experience, or approaches based on pathophysiological principles alone. This approach distinguishes practitioners of EBM from doctors who unquestioningly base their practice on personal experience, expert opinion and authority, or simply tradition – 'the way we've always done this'.

However, it is very important to remember that EBM is not about basing your practice only on RCTs. There may not be an RCT that relates to the issue for your patient so you may have to use evidence from lower down the hierarchy (while recognising its limitations). And of course, things other than *mathematical estimates of the chance of benefit and the risk of harm* will be very important in shaping your practice. These include the views of your patients on the significance of those benefits and harms for them, their personal situations and the cost-effectiveness of the different options, since money spent on one patient cannot be used for the care of a different patient (Barber, 1995). EBM is about using the best available evidence to *guide* your practice.

ACTIVITY 3.2 WHY MIGHT AN RCT WHICH RELATES TO YOUR CLINICAL PROBLEM NOT BE AVAILABLE?

Think about why an RCT might not be a suitable or feasible way of investigating some research questions. Make a list of reasons, and compare your answers with those of some colleagues.

There are a number of possible reasons why an RCT might not be suitable or feasible, and you can find some discussion of this in an article by Nick Black (1996) in the *British Medical Journal* (BMJ). Good reasons that you might have suggested include:

- Ethics: for example, it would not be ethical to conduct an RCT on the safety of a drug in pregnancy or breastfeeding, or the risk of lung cancer and heart disease from smoking.

- Practicality: for example, it might not be feasible to recruit enough people with a very rare condition for an RCT to be big enough to give a reliable answer. (It would also be unethical to recruit people to a study which can't reliably answer its research question.)

- Expense: for example, any difference in the effects on cardiovascular risk between two statins at equivalent lipid-lowering doses is likely to be very small, if it exists at all. To detect such a difference reliably, an RCT would have to recruit many thousands of participants and run for many years: the expense involved would be enormous and could not be justified for the value of the research question.

How do people make decisions?

As a doctor, you will have to make a great many decisions. In this book we are thinking about choosing whether or not to prescribe, and if so, what drug and dose to choose. But the same principles apply to other medical (and non-medical) decisions: although the evidence should inform your decision, it doesn't tell you – or your patient – what to do. You still have to make a decision.

That decision requires you to recall, interpret and apply large volumes of information. Humans use the same processes to handle all large volumes of complex information (Maskrey *et al.*, 2009a).

ACTIVITY 3.3 MAKING DECISIONS

Think about a reasonably important decision you have made recently – something more than what to have for tea! You might think about how you decided where to go on holiday, where to go for an elective or for Foundation Year training, what car or smart phone to buy, or similar.

Think about what things you considered when you were making this decision, and how you got the information you needed.

Compare your answer with a friend. How similar or different were the types of things you considered and the sources you used?

When we have asked this question in workshops, people have always responded in the same way. So, for example, buying a new car: you probably would read a few reviews from trusted sources (on the internet or in a magazine) and talk to some people – perhaps those who already have the car(s) you are thinking of buying but especially people you see as being knowledgeable about cars. You probably wouldn't read lots of detailed technical information, such as the full study reports of the European New Car Assessment Programme or the Society of Automotive Engineers.

Your decision probably came down to a few key factors such as practical needs (a two-seater sports car is no good if you have to tow a horse box or transport a large family), running costs (can you afford the fuel costs and insurance?), safety and reliability, and personal factors such as colour of the car.

When faced with a large quantity of information – whether in a clinical setting or in everyday life – we usually truncate the portion we actually use so as to make a 'good enough' decision. This is known as 'satisficing' (Maskrey *et al.*, 2009a).

Dual-process theory

There are two broad processes which human beings use to make decisions. The one which we all tend to favour is known as system 1 processing. This is unconscious, and involves the construction and use of mental maps and patterns, shortcuts and rules of thumb. These are usually based on brief written summaries, personal experience and talking to colleagues and seeing what they do. Once established, they are very resistant to change (Croskerry, 2009; Gabbay and le May, 2004).

System 1 is very fast and works on pattern recognition. For example, if you saw a child with neck stiffness, photophobia and a non-blanching, petechial rash, we are sure you would make a presumptive diagnosis of meningococcal septicaemia and recognise that the child needed urgent intravenous antibiotics. You would do that very quickly, probably without even being aware of the process you went through to reach those decisions. The alternative – system 2 processing – is much more time-consuming and effortful. It involves a careful, rational analysis and evaluation of all the available information. In this example, it might involve looking up the rash in a textbook, and certainly involves a lot of conscious thought.

The preference we all have for system 1 processing means that we can all too easily ignore things which don't quite fit the pattern. When using system 1, we need to stop and think to check we haven't ignored something important.

Neither system 1 nor system 2 should be regarded as 'good' or 'bad'. System 1 processing can provide life-saving decisions very quickly, as in the example of meningococcal septicaemia above. On the other hand, system 2 processing can locate information which enables us to make a decision when we can't do so using system 1. However, system 2 processing takes more time and this may not be consistent with the pace required of clinical practice.

Although we can make mistakes in system 2, it is in system 1 that our unconscious cognitive biases reside. There is a risk if we develop a pattern of knowledge which we rely on for decisions using only system 1. We need to activate a system 2 check (which could be as simple as checking that, for example, the person with suspected meningococcal septicaemia is not allergic to the proposed antibiotic). Perhaps the most dangerous bias is the blind-spot bias: 'My colleagues are susceptible to these biases, but I'm not.'

Researchers explored how primary care clinicians make decisions about healthcare. Their study was set in two general practices, one in the south of England and the other in the north of England, and used standard methods (non-participant observation, semistructured interviews and documentary review) to collect data over a 2-year time period (Gabbay and le May, 2004).

When analysed, these data showed that clinicians rarely accessed, appraised and used explicit evidence directly from research or other formal sources; rare exceptions were when they might consult such sources after dealing with a case that had particularly challenged them. The authors say that:

> [Clinicians] relied on what we have called 'mindlines'; collectively reinforced, internalised tacit guidelines, which were informed by brief reading, but mainly by their interactions with each other and with opinion leaders, patients, and pharmaceutical representatives and by other sources of largely tacit knowledge that built on their early training and their own and their colleagues' experience.
>
> (Gabbay and le May, 2004, p. 1015)

Think about your practice and the practice you see around you. How often do you see mindlines operating (the mental shortcuts and rules of thumb we talked about as being key characteristics of system 1 processing)? What are the pros and cons of being influenced by colleagues?

A major challenge for you as a doctor will be to pick out the information you need to inform your practice from the almost daily flood of information you receive (see below). However, even if you succeed in this, the preference all humans have for system 1 processing makes it hard to modify practice in the light of new information which conflicts with our previous (perhaps tacit) assumptions and knowledge (Maskrey *et al.*, 2009a).

Shared decision making

You have probably noticed that the old idea of 'doctor knows best' doesn't sit easily with contemporary ideas. Instead, shared decision making, involving patients and professionals together, is increasingly recognised as an essential part of modern healthcare (Marshall and Bibby, 2011). Look back at the definition of EBM by Sackett *et al.* Involving patients in decision making is an integral part of that idea.

A study of patients in seven general practices in London in 2007 found that 39% wanted their GPs to share the decision and 16% wanted to be the main (14%) or only (2%) decision maker themselves. Of the remainder, just 17% wanted the GP to be the only decision maker regarding their care (Cox *et al.*, 2007). GPs underestimated patients' preference for involvement in 23% of the consultations studied. In a survey conducted by the Picker Institute in 2006, 45% of primary care patients who responded indicated that they had not had sufficient involvement in choosing their medication (Picker Institute Europe, 2007).

> **ACTIVITY 3.4 SHARED DECISION MAKING**
>
> Look up the National Institute for Health and Care Excellence (NICE) clinical guideline 76: Medicines adherence: Involving patients in decisions about prescribed medicines and supporting adherence (go to www.nice.org.uk) and see what it recommends about involving patients in decisions about their medicines. Make brief notes on the key principles. When you next have the chance to observe a clinician (such as a doctor, nurse, pharmacist or other healthcare professional) talking with a patient about his or her treatment, compare what the clinician does with the recommendations from NICE. If you can, discuss the interaction with the clinician – and perhaps the patient.

How could you involve patients more in decisions about their medicines? What possible barriers are there and how might you overcome them?

Information management and information mastery

Whether you are a medical student, a Foundation Year doctor, specialist trainee or a consultant or GP principal, you face a constant flood of newly published research, guidance and opinion. This presents a major challenge in identifying not only the important new information you need, but also what now turns out to be wrong or out of date among what you already know (Shaughnessy and Slawson, 1999).

As we have seen, to cope with large volumes of information, we all usually 'satisfice'. However, the strategies many people adopt to manage information carry risks. Many practitioners use expert opinion as a shortcut to information and its application to practice, but evidence reminds us that experts can be wrong and that we need to be cautious when relying on a colleague's advice (Schaafsma *et al.*, 2005).

> **What's the evidence?**
>
> A study conducted among Dutch occupational health physicians compared the accuracy of advice obtained from experts with the best evidence from the literature (Schaafsma *et al.*, 2005). Fourteen occupational physicians were presented with case vignettes and asked to consult with experts of their choice for their advice. The occupational physicians consulted 75 different experts. Overall, expert advice was slightly more likely to be wrong than right: 53% (95% confidence interval (CI) 42–65%) of it was not in line with the published evidence. In 18 cases (24%) the experts explicitly referred to up-to-date research literature. This advice was substantially less likely to be incorrect (17%) than advice that had not mentioned the literature as a source (65%) (difference 48%, 95% CI 27–69%).

How do you use information and advice from colleagues and experts? Slawson and Shaughnessy suggested the following approach:

Using expert-based information

- Determine the level of evidence supporting recommendations – is the recommendation based on patient-oriented or disease-oriented evidence (see Box 3.2 below for the difference)?
- Do not make your own clinical rules out of patient-specific recommendations made by consultants
- Remember the lag time between fact finding and publication
- Realise that authors of reviews and textbooks and speakers at educational conferences often begin with their predetermined conclusions and then find evidence to support only this point of view
- Wisdom gained through experience helps clinicians diagnose disease and perform procedures. Experience is not adequate to remain proficient in treatments: proficiency also requires a knowledge of the medical literature and the ability to think critically with an open mind.

(Slawson and Shaughnessy, 1997, p. 947)

Using what we know about decision making to practise in an evidence-based way

It would be nice to think you could be up to date with the evidence base for a wide range of conditions, but for conditions you see rarely, this is unrealistic. No one could reasonably expect GPs to know 'off the top of their head' how to manage homozygous familial hyperlipidaemia (with an incidence of about 1 case per million), but any parent would expect a GP to be up to date in managing otitis media without having to look things up, because this is a very common condition in primary care. In this example, to make best use of system 1 processing, the GP will assimilate all the up-to-date information required for expert diagnosis and management of otitis media into a mental map and mindline (see section on dual-process theory, above). The GP can then activate this for efficient, effective care.

Information mastery describes a system by which you, as a busy student or doctor, can optimise your system 1 processing and keep it up to date. You will also be able to use system 2 processing effectively and efficiently when this is appropriate – and recognise when this is so (Slawson *et al.*, 1994; Maskrey *et al.*, 2009b). There are three complementary components – foraging, hot-synching and hunting – and you need to use all of them.

Foraging

Many doctors have what we call 'guilt stacks' – piles of journals which have not been opened, or perhaps have not even made it out of their plastic wrappers, but which they hope to try to read 'some day'. Do you?

If you have such a pile, throw it away (or better still, recycle it). There simply isn't time to keep up to date by reading journal articles: there are too many published all the time. Even if you manage to read one article, how do you know there aren't 20 others you haven't read that say the opposite? You need a better system for staying up to date – in other words, an effective foraging service. That is, a service that surveys the literature (and other important sources of information) and alerts you to new information which is both important and likely to be useful to you. Ideally, a good foraging service will place the new evidence in the context of the rest of the evidence base (Slawson *et al.*, 1994).

We saw previously that brief reading is an important shaper of the mindlines which are a key player in system 1 processing. So, a good foraging service will help ensure your mindlines are up to date and in keeping with current evidence.

Case Study 3.1

Foraging also, importantly, helps clinicians identify when they need to activate their system 2 processing. For example, a prescriber (DR) was made aware of the results of the ADDITION-Europe study (Griffin *et al.*, 2011) through a foraging service. This looked at the effect of early intensive multifactorial management (of HbA_{1c}, blood pressure, cholesterol and prescription of aspirin) on 5-year cardiovascular outcomes in people with newly diagnosed type 2 diabetes that had been detected by screening. Although some small reductions in disease-oriented outcomes (HbA_{1c}, blood pressure, total and low-density lipoprotein cholesterol) were seen with intensive management compared with usual care, no statistically significant differences were found in any patient-oriented cardiovascular outcome (i.e. whether patients lived longer or better).

DR had previously assumed that the best approach would be one of 'hitting newly diagnosed type 2 diabetes hard and fast', especially blood glucose control. DR's foraging service highlighted the results of the ADDITION-Europe study and put it in context with other high-quality RCTs, which showed that lowering blood glucose beyond moderate levels had little benefit and could be harmful. This stimulated DR to ask questions to help direct his professional development, including 'What is the value of screening for type 2 diabetes?' and 'What is the value of intensive interventions in type 2 diabetes?'

Why not read the ADDITION-Europe study yourself and see if it challenges your thinking about type 2 diabetes?

Hot-synching

This leads to the second element of information mastery, called hot-synching. You probably have an MP3 player. You need to hot-synch this with your computer periodically to update your playlists. In the same way, you can hot-synch your mind with the evidence you need to know to be able to manage the conditions you see commonly. Most people can only devote about an hour a week to continuing professional development. Instead of unfocused reading or going to lectures on interesting but rare conditions, you can spend this time reviewing summaries of evidence produced by trusted, public-sector organisations (or those with a public-sector ethos) covering just the conditions you see commonly.

Hot-synching is realistic for busy doctors, and fits with the human dimensions of information acquisition and decision making. By facilitating targeted, focused 'offline' system 2 processing, you can continue to use the rapid and efficient system 1 processing in the healthcare setting because your mindlines are based on the best available evidence. Moreover, an effective foraging service, such as the Medicines Information Awareness Service offered by NICE (www.nice.org.uk/mpc/MedicinesPrescribingAlerts.jsp) will alert you to new, important information published since you last hot-synched on a particular topic (Maskrey et al., 2009b).

Hunting

In addition to foraging and hot-synching, you need an approach to finding information when you don't have what you need in your (now evidence-based) mindlines and mental maps – in other words, when you are stuck. This third element of information mastery is called hunting, and supports system 2 processing. It is an approach which enables you to find useful information rapidly when you need it, and also enables you to know that you have found the *best* available answer there is, not just *an* answer whose only merit is that you found it easily (Slawson et al., 1994). It is a much more directed and refined approach than simply searching Medline or Google Scholar and we'll explain more below.

What is useful information?

The information that is likely to be the best – that is, the most useful – that clinicians can find, whether through foraging, hot-synching or hunting, is expressed in the usefulness equation (Box 3.1) (Slawson et al., 1994; Maskrey et al., 2009b). This is simply saying that a piece of information which is both highly relevant and highly valid and which is found easily and quickly is likely to be extremely useful. That same piece of information would be less useful if a great deal of work was required to find it. Equally, a piece of information which is readily available but is either not very relevant or not very valid is also not very useful. In fact it might be positively unhelpful.

Box 3.1 Usefulness of a piece of information (adapted from Slawson et al., 1994)

Usefulness of a piece of clinical information $= \dfrac{\text{relevance}^{a} \times \text{validity}^{b}}{\text{work required}^{c}}$

a Information that is likely to be relevant to front-line care includes that which relates to a feasible intervention and which shows a direct effect on whether patients live longer or better (see Box 3.2).

---

b   The information's validity depends on factors such as study design, statistical power and attempts to minimise bias and confounding.

c   This is the work required to find the information and, by extension, the work required to establish its relevance and validity.

Relevance before validity

With a little practice, assessing the relevance of a piece of information is quick and easy – it can usually be done from the abstract alone and most of the time it takes only a few seconds – so it's best to screen for relevance first. The FOCC mnemonic helpfully reminds us of the key things to consider (Box 3.2: Slawson *et al.*, 1994).

Box 3.2 Screening for relevance: the FOCC mnemonic (adapted from Slawson *et al.*, 1994)

Feasible: Is the intervention feasible in my clinical practice?

Outcomes: Does the study report patient-oriented outcomes?*

Common: Is the condition or clinical situation common in my clinical practice?

Change: Might I have to change my practice if this information turns out to be valid and is in keeping with the rest of the evidence base?

*A patient-oriented outcome is an outcome which is directly important to patients. Examples include a reduction in the rate of heart attacks and strokes, a reduction in the risk of developing diabetic foot ulcers or a reduction in night-time awakenings in people with asthma. This is in contrast to disease-oriented outcomes: these do not directly tell us if the intervention helps patients to live longer or live better. They are surrogate markers and are often laboratory tests. Examples include changes in blood pressure, HbA_{1C} in type 2 diabetes and peak expiratory flow volume in asthma. These may be useful surrogate measures, which indicate improvements for patients, but equally they may not, and indeed can sometimes mislead.

Unless you can say 'yes' to each of the criteria in the FOCC mnemonic, it is extremely unlikely to be relevant to you. You can simply say, 'I don't know, and I don't care'. At most, read it for interest – but don't think it will help you keep up to date or answer a clinical question (Slawson *et al.*, 1994).

ACTIVITY 3.5 SCREENING FOR RELEVANCE

With some colleagues, scan through the current editions of the BMJ, *The Lancet*, the *New England Journal of Medicine*, or similar 'ivy league' general medical journals to which you have access. Apply the FOCC criteria to each article, and see for how many of them you can say 'yes' to each FOCC criterion.

Are you surprised?

How do your answers compare with your colleagues' answers?

We find that doctors most often have difficulty applying the 'outcome' criterion: remember, the question is: 'Does this study tell me directly if the treatment helped patients live longer or better?' So changes in blood pressure, or peak flow, or similar measures don't count. We need to see outcomes such as mortality rates, rates of admission to hospital and improvements in quality of life scores.

Whether foraging, hot-synching or hunting, we need to use the information mastery pyramid (Figure 3.1: Slawson *et al.*, 1994; Maskrey *et al.*, 2009b). This is different from a hierarchy of evidence, because it is for a different purpose.

The pyramid is ranked in descending order of usefulness. The most useful information sources are at the top of the pyramid. When hunting for information, you need to drill down from the top to find the information you need. If you find an answer in the sources towards the top of the pyramid, this is likely to be the best answer available: you can stop drilling (Slawson *et al.*, 1994). If a resource has NICE accreditation (www.nice.org.uk/aboutnice/accreditation/index.jsp), such as guidance from NICE, Scottish Intercollegiate Guidelines Network (SIGN) and the Medicines and Healthcare Products Regulatory Agency, you can be confident that processes used to create it are robust and reliable. A key feature of the information mastery approach to using high-quality information to inform practice is that someone other than busy front-line practitioners – preferably a trusted public-sector organisation or one with a similar ethos – does the selection and critical appraisal.

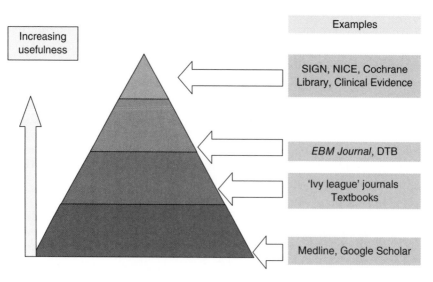

Figure 3.1 The information mastery pyramid. SIGN, Scottish Intercollegiate Guidelines Network; NICE, National Institute for Health and Care Excellence; DTB, *Drug and Therapeutics Bulletin*. (Adapted from Slawson *et al.*, 1994.)

At the top of the pyramid, NICE-accredited sources such as NICE and SIGN guidance are based on syntheses of all the available evidence, which has been systematically searched for and rigorously appraised. They are likely to be the most useful sources, most often, because their validity is high and the work you need to do to access them and extract information is low. They provide recommendations for practice which will address most clinical situations, so they are most likely to be relevant. Similarly, the Cochrane Library, Clinical Evidence, and similar synthesised sources of information, produced by trusted and trustworthy providers of information in a timely and up-to-date manner, are likely to be more useful to busy doctors than sources further down the pyramid.

Next come sources such as the *Drug and Therapeutics Bulletin*, which publishes high-quality evidence-based reviews, and the *EBM Journal*, which scans other journals, assesses the validity of evidence presented in them, summarises this and provides a commentary.

'Ivy league' journals, such as the BMJ, *The Lancet* and the *New England Journal of Medicine*, come next. The quality of their content is usually high, but you need some critical appraisal skills to assess the articles' validity properly, and many articles will not be relevant. Textbooks are easier to access, but the validity may not be so high: they may present information selectively and the information may be out of date.

Medline and Google Scholar and similar sources at the bottom will provide lots of information, but the usefulness is quite low, because a lot of work is required to filter out the relevant and valid information.

Is this piece of evidence valid?

Screening for validity is more difficult and requires some expertise and also time and frequent practice. There are lots of ways in which you can acquire and develop these basic skills. However, you don't have to be an expert in critical appraisal – it is reasonably easy to spot the more common fatal flaws. We have space here only to indicate the kind of things you need to know and we recommend you do further study (Activity 3.6, below).

Is it a high level of evidence?

As we said earlier, whenever possible you should base decisions on evidence from high-quality RCTs or systematic reviews and meta-analyses of high-quality RCTs. However, such evidence is not always available and it may be necessary to use less robust evidence, such as observational studies, recognising their potential limitations.

Is the result statistically significant?

The probability that the difference observed is due to the play of chance is indicated by the *p* value. By convention, if a result could occur by chance less than one time in 20 (or 5 in 100, $p = 0.05$) then that result is accepted as proven 'beyond reasonable doubt' and said to be 'statistically significant'. 'No statistically significant difference' does not necessarily mean there is truly no difference between the interventions – that might be so, or it might be that the study is underpowered (see below).

Is the result clinically important?

It is possible for a study to produce a highly statistically significant result which has very limited clinical value. For example, a difference in time to walk 50 metres might be reduced by a highly statistically significant extent (say, $p = 0.001$) by one treatment compared to another, but in absolute terms the difference might be only a few seconds, or even less.

What do the numbers mean?

There will be a key expression of difference in the results – relative risk, relative risk reduction, absolute risk reduction, odds ratio or hazard ratio, numbers needed to treat (NNT) or harm (NNH). There is no shortcut to developing the skills required to understand what those terms mean, but this is an essential skill for modern medicine.

ACTIVITY 3.6 WHAT DO THE NUMBERS MEAN?

You may well have seen clopidogrel co-prescribed with aspirin to people who have had an episode of acute coronary syndrome. The key evidence for this comes from the CURE study (The Clopidogrel in Unstable Angina to Prevent Recurrent Events (CURE) Trial Investigators, 2001).

In the study, 12,562 patients who had presented within 24 hours of the onset of symptoms were randomly assigned to receive clopidogrel (300mg immediately, followed by 75mg once daily) or placebo for 3–12 months. Both groups also received aspirin 75–325mg daily. The primary outcome – a composite of death from cardiovascular causes, non-fatal myocardial infarction or stroke – occurred in 9.3% of the patients in the clopidogrel plus aspirin group and 11.4% of the patients in the placebo plus aspirin group (relative risk 0.80; 95% CI, 0.72–0.90; $p < 0.001$). More patients in the clopidogrel plus aspirin group developed major bleeding than in the placebo plus aspirin group (3.7% versus 2.7%; relative risk 1.38, 95% CI 1.13–1.67; $p = 0.001$), but there was no significant difference in the number of life-threatening bleeds (2.1% versus 1.8%, $p = 0.13$).

For the primary outcome and the outcome of major bleeds, calculate:

- the relative risk reduction or increase;
- the absolute risk reduction or increase;
- the NNT or NNH.

Explain what is indicated by the *p* values and 95% confidence intervals.

How would you explain to a patient how taking aspirin plus clopidogrel instead of aspirin alone would affect the chances of avoiding a major cardiovascular event and having a major bleed?

If you are having difficulty with this, look at the BMJ learning module on 'Understanding statistics' and/or the National Prescribing Centre website (both of which use the example of clopidogrel and the CURE study): see the Going Further section, below.

Were there enough people in the study for long enough?

If the study was too small, or lasted for too short a period, or the outcome of interest occurred too infrequently, the study may not have been able to say that an observed difference between treatments was statistically significant, even if the result wasn't just due to chance and the difference really exists. Such studies are said to be underpowered.

Was the allocation concealed?

You don't have to understand the details of allocation concealment to know that it is important, but in essence the study investigators should not know to which group potential subjects would be assigned before enrolling them. It is not the same as blinding, but is in fact a potential source of recruitment bias. Trials with unconcealed allocation consistently overestimate benefit by about 40%. Trial reports should either say that allocation was concealed, or describe an allocation method which assured this (for example, contacting a distant allocation service by telephone to assign patients to treatment after they have been enrolled).

ACTIVITY 3.7 HOW DO YOU MAKE DECISIONS IN YOUR DAILY PRACTICE?

Take some time to reflect critically on the decisions you made in the course of a typical day. How much thinking, and what type of thinking, went on for each decision – or indeed, did you just 'know' what to do (system 1)? Why not discuss a day's notes with a colleague?

What were these decisions based on – what you knew to be the evidence, what you thought to be the evidence, or what someone else – with all the same cognitive biases as any human – said was the evidence?

Probably the aspect of information mastery and decision making in which most medical students and doctors can make most progress most quickly is the adoption of an effective hot-synching system. You can follow this up by investigating one or more foraging tools. There are many available, and the resources in the Going Further section below can help identify those best suited to your needs. Above all, you are likely to find that seeking out colleagues who want to try a similar approach to better information management and better decision making is extremely helpful in putting these ideas into practice.

Chapter summary

A large part of your job as a doctor is to make decisions. This in turn requires you to identify, recall, interpret and apply large volumes of information. This chapter has focused on two important components of this: firstly, how people – health professionals and patients alike – make decisions and how these decisions might be made better; and secondly, it offers an approach to managing the large volumes of information with which doctors are faced almost daily.

GOING FURTHER

Black N (1996) Why we need observational studies to evaluate the effectiveness of health care. *British Medical Journal*, 312: 1215–1218.

British Medical Journal learning zone (see especially 'understanding statistics' and 'understanding statistics 2'): http://learning.bmj.com/learning/home.html

Dr Chris Cates' EBM website:

- Main site: www.nntonline.net;
- VisualRx (generates Cates plots): www.nntonline.net/visualrx

EBM Journal (provides useful, high-quality summaries of evidence: helpful for hunting): http://ebm.bmj.com

Information Centre for Health and Social Care (2011) *Use of NICE Appraised Medicines in the NHS in England – 2009, Experimental statistics.* Leeds: ICHSC.

National Prescribing Centre (NPC)*

- Online video: *Making decisions better.* www.npc.nhs.uk/evidence/making_decisions_better/making_decisions_better.php
- eLearning resources on evidence-informed decision making: www.npc.nhs.uk/evidence/index.php
- Online video on using patient decision aids (PDAs): www.npc.nhs.uk/patient_decision_aids/pda_movie/patient_decision_aids.php
- Directory of NPC-produced PDAs and further information about PDAs: www.npc.nhs.uk/patient_decision_aids/pda.php

Tufts University School of Medicine (Department of Family Medicine) Center for Information Mastery: http://medicine.tufts.edu/Education/Academic-Departments/Clinical-Departments/Family-Medicine/Center-for-Information-Mastery

---

*Note: following the integration of the NPC into NICE, as the NICE Medicines and Prescribing Centre, the npc.nhs.uk site is now a legacy website. The extensive catalogue of materials will still be available to view and download for as long as the information contained within them remains accurate and up to date. They will be updated in due course.

chapter 4

Working with **Others**

Greg Heath and Helen Bradbury

Achieving your medical degree

This chapter will help you meet the following requirements of *Tomorrow's Doctors* (General Medical Council (GMC), 2009):

22. Learn and work effectively within a multi-professional team.

    (a) Understand and respect the roles and expertise of health and social care professionals in the context of working and learning as a multi-professional team.

    (b) Understand the contribution that effective interdisciplinary teamworking makes to the delivery of safe and high-quality care.

    (c) Work with colleagues in ways that best serve the interests of the patients, passing on information and handing over care, demonstrating flexibility, adaptability and a problem-solving approach.

It will also link to *Good Medical Practice* (GMC, 2013a)

and

Good Practice in Prescribing and Managing Medicines and Devices (GMC, 2013b), particularly paragraphs 12–13 and 30–43.

Chapter overview

Good communication is key for effective teamwork. A single patient may be cared for by a multitude of professionals. While some of these may form part of the hospital health-care team, others will be located within the local community. In order that patient care is not compromised, every member of the team must collaborate with one another. The aim of this chapter is to encourage you to collaborate interprofessionally to achieve safe and quality patient care. In keeping with the theme of the book, the importance on collaborative working in relation to prescribing will be emphasised. After reading this chapter you will be able to:

- contribute to the multidisciplinary team ensuring safe, effective prescribing for patients;
- define the different roles, responsibilities and expertise of a range of healthcare professionals in the prescribing process;
- work in partnership with colleagues for the benefit of patients.

Introduction

Patients are rarely cared for by a single professional group. More often than not, a plethora of healthcare professionals allied to medicine are involved in their care. Knowledge of such professionals and how they work and their professional standing is key to working effectively within the healthcare team to ensure safe prescribing (Hammick *et al.*, 2009). Bond (2001) has illuminated other key components that correlate positively with effective team working. These are: having a clear understanding of your own role; pooling knowledge, skills and resources; and sharing the responsibility for outcomes.

The interprofessional approach to ensuring the patient receives the appropriate medication involves a heterogeneous group of professionals either in healthcare or the social setting to achieve the patient's needs. These are illustrated in Activities 4.1 and 4.2 (see below). It is not uncommon for each professional group to have different management plans. Thus, in order to mitigate the potential for such disparity, it is vital that the professional groups collaborate to form agreed goals. It is noteworthy that collaboration is an acquired skill and can lead to conflict resolution in order to achieve the desired outcome. The latter may arise as a result of the varying boundaries implemented by the disparate professional groups working within the team. Notwithstanding such challenges, the benefits to the patient are irrefutable.

Roles and responsibilities of healthcare professionals in the prescribing process

ACTIVITY 4.1 THE MEANING OF TERMS

What do you understand by the terms independent prescribing and supplementary prescribing?

Write down your thoughts, discuss them with colleagues and be prepared to come back to them when you have finished reading this chapter and see whether (and how) they have changed.

Supplementary prescribers are authorised to prescribe medicines within an agreed clinical management plan for patients whose condition has been assessed or diagnosed by an independent prescriber. In these terms an independent prescriber is a doctor or dentist. So the supplementary prescriber is responsible for continuing care after an independent medical prescriber has assessed the health of the patient. If the patient's care needs exceed those within the supplementary prescriber's expertise, the practitioner will refer the patient back to his/her independent prescriber.

Non-medical independent prescribers are responsible for the assessment of patients with either diagnosed or undiagnosed conditions and for implementing decisions related to the clinical management of the patient. The non-medical independent prescriber is able to prescribe any medicines as part of the treatment plan.

ACTIVITY 4.2 WHO CAN PRESCRIBE?

List the supplementary and independent prescribers that you are likely to encounter as a doctor.

After you have read the following paragraphs, check back to see whether you have missed any groups or individuals. Had you realised there were so many?

Supplementary prescribers include the following registered practitioners: nurses, pharmacists, midwives, optometrists, radiographers, physiotherapists, chiropodists and podiatrists. This list can be amended from time to time.

Independent prescribers are doctors and dentists. Other prescribers such as nurses, midwives, pharmacists and optometrists are known as non-medical prescribers. You may consider the use of the negative 'non' inappropriate, as all of these individuals care for patients and can prescribe for them. Prescribers can prescribe from an extensive range of medicines and, in the case of nurses, midwives and pharmacists, that range is the full *British National Formulary* (BNF), with some small exceptions. Controlled drugs were excluded or strictly restricted until 2012 when, with very few exceptions, schedule 2–5 controlled drugs were added to the lists of drugs available to prescribe.

Physiotherapists and podiatrists are the next group of professionals who, following accreditation, will be able to acquire independent prescribing status from 2014 onwards.

What's the evidence for expanding the eligibility of prescribing groups?

Prescribing of medicines other than by doctors and dentists was promoted by the government in the late 1990s as part of the modernisation of the NHS. The aims were: first, by increasing the contributions of other healthcare professionals, the needs of the local health economies would be met; second, it would allow the development of more flexible services which, as a consequence, would enable healthcare professionals to provide better care for vulnerable groups, especially those that were geographically difficult to reach; third, it gave patients greater access to medicines, and fourth, it used the skills of professionals such as pharmacists, nurses and midwives more appropriately.

Although the Cumberlege report (DHSS, 1986) was the first document to support nurse prescribing, it was the Crown report (Department of Health, 1998) that advocated the notion that district nurses and health visitors should be allowed to prescribe from a limited formulary.

Some of the notable documents released by the Department of Health leading up to the inception of non-medical prescribing are listed below:

Department of Health (1999) *Making a Difference: Strengthening the nursing, midwifery and health visitor contribution to health and healthcare.*

Department of Health (2000a) *The NHS Plan: A plan for investment, a plan for reform.*

This highlighted the importance of the dissolution of demarcations between clinical roles in enabling professionals to work more flexibly in order to augment patient care.

Department of Health (2000b) *Pharmacy in the Future: Implementing the NHS plan.*

This essentially outlined the delivery of pharmacy services in the UK.

Health and Social Care Act 2001.

This identified the list of potential additional prescribers.

There are three other elements about the supply and administration of medicines which you need to know about in order for you to fully understand the roles, responsibilities and expertise of other healthcare professionals in the prescribing process. These are Patient Group Directions (PGDs), Patient Specific Directions (PSDs) and electronic prescribing.

Patient Group Directions

A PGD is a specific written statement, drawn up locally by doctors and pharmacists, for the supply and administration of medicines by other healthcare professionals in an identified clinical situation (NHS, Patient Group Directions).

There are many individuals who can supply (not prescribe) medicines using a PGD. These include registered:

- pharmacists;
- dietitians;
- midwives;
- health visitors;
- nurses;

- occupational therapists;
- optometrists;
- orthotists and prosthetists;
- speech and language therapists;
- chiropodists;
- orthoptists;
- physiotherapists;
- radiographers;
- paramedics.

The above healthcare professionals can only supply and administer medicines under a PGD as named individuals and must be authorised by the employing organisation. Healthcare assistants cannot work under PGDs because they are not registered nurses.

You may become involved in writing or signing off PGDs. There are many examples now, although when this was first introduced in 2004, each organisation, whether in a primary or secondary care setting, had to draw up its own following guidance given by the Department of Health.

Particular caution should be exercised in any decision to draw up PGDs relating to antibiotics. Microbial resistance is a public health matter of major importance and great care should be taken to ensure that the inclusion of antibiotics in a direction is absolutely necessary and will not jeopardise strategies to combat increasing resistance. You would be expected to involve a local microbiologist in drawing up this type of PGD. Other areas where a specialist may become involved in drawing up PGDs are family planning, physiotherapy and supplying medicines for young children.

Exemptions

Midwives, chiropodists/podiatrists, optometrists and paramedics, for example, have specific exemptions in medicines legislation to supply or administer medicines. Provided the requirements of any conditions attaching to those exemptions are met, a PGD is not required. For example, registered podiatrists have exemptions under medicines legislation for parenteral administration of a number of prescription-only medicines, including bupivacaine and lignocaine.

Patient Specific Directions

A PSD is a written instruction from an independent prescriber once the patient has been assessed. It allows another healthcare professional to supply or administer a medicine to a specified patient or several named patients (e.g. clinic list). Generally it is a direct instruction and does not require a healthcare professional to assess the patient.

Electronic prescribing

As you are well aware, central to modern medicine is the issue, where appropriate, of a prescription. This needs to be done in a timely manner, giving patients easy access to their medicines and appliances. As we have said in Chapter 1, good communication between prescriber and patients is essential and for prescription services to work efficiently there also needs to be good communication with pharmacists, dispensing doctors or appliance manufacturers. Electronic prescription services allow digitally signed prescriptions to be transmitted electronically from primary care prescribers to be stored on a server, from which they can be downloaded and dispensed.

The team

Since the reason for working collaboratively is to optimise the care of your patients, they should be included as an integral member of your team (see Chapter 1), so your team is truly patient-centred.

One of the criticisms of the new working pattern, resulting partly from the European Working Time Directive, is the dissolution of the 'medical firms'. Traditionally, such 'firms' consisted of at least one consultant, specialist registrar and several juniors. Owing to the new working shift pattern, junior doctors, in particular, are incorporated in more than one team. This underscores the importance of communicating well with others in order that important information is not omitted (see section on handover later in this chapter). Primary or community practice-based teams are however relatively static, which gives them a major advantage over their hospital counterparts with regard to maintaining continuity of patient care.

Collaborative practice

The World Health Organization suggests how collaborative practice happens in its *Framework for Action on Interprofessional Action and Collaborative Practice*:

> *when multiple health workers from different professional backgrounds work together with patients, families, carers and communities to deliver the highest quality of care. It allows health workers to engage any individual whose skills can help achieve local health goals.*

(World Health Organization, 2010)

In 2012, the National Prescribing Centre, on behalf of the National Institute for Health and Clinical Excellence (NICE: recently renamed National Institute for Health and Care Excellence), published a single competency framework for all practitioners. Its purpose is to consolidate the profession-specific prescribing frameworks in order to provide a single common framework for any prescriber regardless of professional background (National Prescribing Centre, 2012). In short, the framework is divided into three domains: domain A relates to the competencies specific to the consultation, such as knowledge and shared decision making; domain B illuminates the competencies attributed to effective, safe prescribing; finally, domain C highlights the competencies needed for prescribing in context and highlights the importance of collaborating with other prescribing colleagues; see Box 4.1.

Box 4.1 National Prescribing Centre competency relating to self and others

Competency 9: Self and others

Works in partnership with colleagues for the benefit of patients. Is self-aware and confident in own ability as a prescriber.

68. Thinks and acts as part of a multidisciplinary team to ensure that continuity of care is developed and not compromised.

69. Establishes relationships with other professionals based on understanding, trust and respect for each other's roles in relation to prescribing.

70. Recognises and deals with pressures that might result in inappropriate prescribing (for example, pharmaceutical industry, media, patient, colleagues).

71. Negotiates the appropriate level of support and supervision for role as prescriber.

72. Provides support and advice to other prescribers where appropriate.

Interprofessional education

The GMC's document *Tomorrow's Doctors* (2009) clearly states that newly qualified doctors should be cognisant of the roles of other healthcare professionals. The concept of interprofessional education, whereby students/professionals learn with, from and about each other, has been embraced by an increasing number of medical schools and postgraduate institutions in order to improve collaboration (CAIPE, 2002). One aim of exposing medical students to allied healthcare professionals and their undergraduate counterparts before they work together is to enhance the knowledge of their respective roles, which will thus lead to early collaboration in patient care.

In the adaptation of Thistlethwaite and Moran's (2010) literature review, Thistlethwaite (2011) divides interprofessional learning outcomes into six categories:

1. teamwork;
2. roles and responsibilities;
3. communication;
4. learning/reflection;
5. the patient;
6. ethical/attitudes.

Teamwork

You as the practitioner are expected to act as an effective team member possessing the requisite knowledge of skills and attitudes. In addition, you should, where appropriate, assume the roles and responsibilities of team leader and team member. Although you may be a junior doctor, you may have medical students in your team allowing you to adopt a leadership role.

As a newly qualified doctor, you will encounter numerous healthcare professionals who will be able to provide you with help and advice regarding the management of your patient. As alluded to earlier, some of the nurses that you may be working with will be specialists in their field and possess independent prescribing status: for example, cardiology nurses prescribing warfarin in the atrial fibrillation clinics. Others may adopt a supplementary prescribing role and seek your advice when the patient's condition deteriorates so as to fall out of the remit of the approved treatment plan. It remains incumbent on you, as the prescriber, to seek senior advice whether from a doctor or other independent prescriber if you are unsure as to the best advice to give in the latter situation.

Roles and responsibilities

It is vital that you are conversant with the different roles, responsibilities and expertise of your colleagues and are aware of professional boundaries. Negative stereotypes of other professionals may have an inhibitory effect on the ability for individuals to learn with, from and about each other. This has been highlighted by the study of Tunstall-Pedoe et al. (2003), in which medical students were deemed to possess more hubris than their nursing contemporaries and, as a consequence, to be less considerate towards them. Challenging misconceptions in relation to professional roles is therefore important and will lead to a more harmonious relationship.

Another professional group who are an important part of the team are pharmacists. They are highly knowledgeable in their field, and, as such, will be able to provide you with invaluable advice when prescribing medicines. Examples include advising on drug choice, highlighting the potential for drug interactions, recommending drug doses and delivery and ensuring that antibiotics are prescribed according to hospital guidelines. Moreover, pharmacists commonly acquire the drug history from the patient and often verify the prescriptions from the patient's GP and another source. This is called medicines reconciliation. Thus, when acquiring a drug history from a patient who has forgotten his or her prescription and is unable to recall the medications that are habitually administered, it is prudent to prescribe only those medications that necessitate immediate management of the patient's condition until a history is obtained from a reliable source. This reduces the propensity towards prescribing errors and their potential consequences. Pharmacy technicians are indispensable in this regard in addition to ensuring that medications are provided on the ward.

Communication

Effective communication between practitioners and patients is positively correlated with patient health outcomes (Stewart, 1995), improvements in patient satisfaction (Williams *et al.*, 1998) and adherence to treatment regimen (DiMatteo, 2004). Conversely, healthcare professionals' failure to communicate effectively within a multidisciplinary team may have a negative impact on a patient's well-being (Gittell *et al.*, 2000).

In order to communicate effectively, you should have mechanisms in place to ensure that patients' essential clinical information is disseminated clearly and that it is handed over at the beginning and end of shifts (see later). Electronic discharge summaries are utilised in the majority of hospitals within the UK and, when written in the way they are intended, provide clear information relating to the patient's admission, particularly in relation to medication changes.

Finally, as a result of working in a multidisciplinary team, there will be times when you may not agree with a colleague's opinion or you may have reservations about the behaviour of certain members of the team. The ability to negotiate and resolve conflicts is an important skill to acquire and it is vital that you know who to approach in order to ameliorate such events should they arise. From a prescribing perspective, if you have doubts relating to the appropriateness of a colleague's prescribing then you must liaise with a senior colleague (ideally one pertaining to the prescribing role in question) in order to mitigate potential harm to the patient and to address any difficulties that your colleague may be having regarding his or her role in the prescribing team.

Learning/reflection

The ability to reflect critically on your relationship with team members is essential to professional development. In addition, critiquing your own preconceived ideas on other professionals should help to avoid stereotyped views.

Unfortunately, we are not immune to making errors. As highlighted by the National Prescribing Centre (2012), one of the competencies relates to the prescriber's ability to strive for improvement. This means reflecting on prescribing errors in order to avoid the risk of further events. Reporting prescribing errors and near misses is actively encouraged. If a colleague fills out an incident reporting form highlighting a prescribing error made by you, do not take it as a criticism. Rather, use this as a learning opportunity. Incident reporting relates to clinical governance, ensuring we offer the best service to our patients. In order that we may learn from our mistakes it is important that we engender a no-blame culture. If you think about it, if we apportion blame on everybody who makes an unintentional error then the incentive to report will be diminished, resulting in a commensurate decline in ameliorating future negative events (see Chapter 7).

Auditing prescriptions provides an excellent method of reflecting how well the team delivers patient care. Presentation of the results should be done in the presence of all members of the healthcare team. Auditing the results with another prescriber (preferably an alternative independent or supplementary prescriber) serves to foster strong professional relationships within the team.

The patient

The patient is central to interprofessional care and all team members should collaborate in the best interests of the patient. This frequently involves other individuals, such as family members or carers. One must recognise the fact that the patient is seen as a partner in the consultation (see Chapter 1).

When prescribing medication, you must respect the patient's values, beliefs and expectations about the medications. In the majority of cases, you will be relying on patients to take responsibility for their medicines and self-manage their conditions. Liaising with other members of the prescribing team is helpful in this regard. For example, pharmacists and pharmacy technicians can demonstrate inhaler techniques for your patient suffering from chronic obstructive airways disease.

Ethical/attitudes

This refers to the fact that one should not only acknowledge the views and ideas of other professionals but also perceive them as equally valid and important.

Handover

Since the implementation of the European Working Time Directive and the reduction in the number of working hours that a doctor is allowed to work, the importance of disseminating important clinical information at the beginning and end of each shift is paramount in providing effective patient care. Unlike the nursing profession, formal handovers are a relatively new concept amongst doctors. Moreover, the handovers involving doctors are rarely interprofessional.

Handovers are usually conducted twice daily: the first occurs in the morning, when the events of the evening are discussed; the second occurs at the end of the evening/beginning of night shifts. The rationale of this process is to transfer the care of the patient to the new, incoming team. Ideally, such transition should be seamless.

There can be significant ramifications related to poorly implemented handovers. Inadequate patient care may lead to life-threatening consequences which in turn may lead to litigation. Other problems as a result of inadequate handovers include:

- wrong diagnoses made or inappropriate investigations requested;
- failure to monitor high-risk treatments;
- failure to avert predicable medical problems (for example, hyperkalaemia in a patient suffering from acute kidney injury);
- failure to act upon abnormalities uncovered by previous investigations;
- failure to prescribe appropriate medications or to omit those having a deleterious effect on the patient.

As mentioned previously, handovers are frequently uniprofessional. However, some departments are encouraging other professionals to attend and this provides the opportunity for the individuals involved to learn from another. It also serves to consolidate the information delivered by the outgoing team. Handovers may take on many guises, ranging from verbal or written communication only to a combination of the two, which is recommended in the literature (Pothier *et al.*, 2005). The propensity to forget salient information is more likely to occur following handovers that involve verbal dissemination of facts alone.

On occasions, your colleagues may have had to attend an emergency elsewhere in the hospital and will be handing over the shift work via the telephone. If this is the case, it is vital that you write down all the information given to you and summarise the information that you have acquired to the referring individual. This gives the opportunity for the referrer to add any additional information that may have been overlooked.

Case Study 4.1

A 70-year-old woman with a history of type 2 diabetes, chronic kidney disease and hypertension was admitted as a result of generalised deterioration. Drugs on admission included ramipril 5mg daily and gliclazide M/R 60mg daily. A urine dipstick was positive for nitrites, leukocytes and protein and she was commenced on trimethoprim together with intravenous fluids and enoxaparin for venous thromboembolism prophylaxis. She had been admitted 48 hours previously and was making little improvement despite the antibiotics.

A microbiologist called at 14.00 and left a message with the healthcare assistant (as all doctors were busy) to say that the infection was resistant to trimethoprim but sensitive to amoxicillin. The message was disseminated to the F1 doctor on the ward who placed the details on his jobs list.

You attend the evening handover at 20.45. The woman in question is not discussed. You are called to see her at 03.00 as she was complaining of chest pain. An electrocardiogram revealed large T waves and reduced p waves, consistent with hyperkalaemia. An urgent blood sample revealed a potassium level of 6.8mmol/L. Her previous potassium level was 5.9mmol/L (upper limit of normal is 5.5mmol/L) on admission (baseline 5.0mmol/L).

What factors contributed to her signs and symptoms?

Two potential factors could be related to her hyperkalaemia. The first question to answer is whether or not she is dehydrated. Signs suggestive of this include reduced skin turgor and low jugular venous pressure.

In the first instance it is important to assess a patient when you acquire the knowledge that he/she is administered an ineffective antibiotic. The patient's potassium was slightly raised on admission, suggesting that it should have been monitored daily, and her angiotensin-converting enzyme (ACE) inhibitor temporarily withdrawn at the outset. It is also advisable to check side-effects of all drugs prescribed for the patient via the BNF. Biochemically, the urea will be disproportionately raised. However, she was commenced on intravenous fluids so one would hope that this was addressed.

The other issue is polypharmacy. Ramipril (an ACE inhibitor), trimethoprim and, to some extent, enoxaparin can all increase potassium levels in the blood. Trimethoprim is often overlooked as a cause of such a metabolic disturbance. Moreover, the patient's urine sample culture results suggest that her infection was resistant to this drug and this should have been dealt with during the afternoon.

This would have been particularly relevant if the patient's urinary tract infection was sensitive to trimethoprim and amoxicillin as the temptation to continue with the former would be significant.

When you look at the drug chart, you notice that a pharmacist has written the admitting potassium value next to the ramipril prescription with a note to monitor the potassium. Pharmacists write this information for a very good reason. The information written should act as an *aide-mémoire* to monitor levels or to change medications in light of the patient's present physical state and should not be ignored.

If you are unable to complete all tasks, those left outstanding should be discussed at handover to allow prioritisation. This emphasises the importance of effective communication during the handover period.

The incident should also be reported to allow reflection of the event both in terms of handover and iatrogenic causes of hyperkalaemia.

Transferring care from the hospital to the community

Many patients, especially those with chronic conditions, will be cared for in both primary (community) and secondary (hospital) settings. To some, their principal carer is their hospital consultant/s; to others, it is their GP with whom they are registered or who they visit most frequently. Not infrequently, specialist nurses are at the forefront of patient care especially in the community, e.g. the support provided by the Macmillan community nurses to patients with cancer. Moreover, as mentioned earlier, from 2012, nurses and pharmacist independent prescribers have been given jurisdiction to prescribe controlled drugs.

In view of the fact that patients may have many professionals involved in the management of their condition/s, it is imperative that you ascertain the details of such in order to maximise continuity of care to ascertain what the patient understands about his/her condition and why. Whilst the patient's understanding may be underpinned by information obtained through the internet, more often than not it is via a healthcare professional. Overtly dismissing these views increases the risk of breaking down your relationship with your patient. If you disagree with the views purported to originate from a particular professional, it is prudent to liaise with the relevant professional to seek clarification. This could be done by yourself, following discussion with a senior colleague, or by the senior colleague. Either way, the importance of working effectively with others is paramount in optimising your patient's well-being.

Discussions with professionals in the community frequently involve the phone as opposed to face to face. The telephone poses particular challenges, especially when language barriers coexist. When confronted with such barriers, for example, seeking clarification of the patient's regular medication from his/her GP, it is important that you politely request for the information to be faxed or emailed. This serves to reduce potential prescribing errors and may allow you to establish a cause for the patient's complaint if it is related to a side-effect of a particular drug being administered.

The responsibility of prescribing lies with the prescriber and this should be borne in mind when you are discharging patients. It is therefore imperative that you foster close links with the nursing staff in addition to the pharmacists on your ward. When discharging patients on new medications, it is important that you disseminate this information clearly to the GP in the discharge summary. Furthermore, any medication that may require monitoring for specific side-effects, such as amiodarone, or that requires therapeutic monitoring in the community, such as warfarin, should be made explicit in your communication.

ACTIVITY 4.3 PREPARING A PATIENT FOR DISCHARGE

Your patient was diagnosed with type 2 diabetes 20 years ago and was admitted under your team with sepsis secondary to pneumonia. She recovered well with intravenous (IV) co-amoxiclav and oral clarithromycin antibiotics. Her medicines on admission were ramipril 5mg daily, metformin 750mg twice a day and simvastatin 40mg daily.

However, as a result of her infection, her kidney function has deteriorated and your consultant advises stopping her ramipril (temporarily) and metformin (permanently) as her blood glucose levels were consistently high at 20mmol/L. She has been assessed by the diabetic team, who commenced her on insulin: Insulin Mixtard 30 20 units subcutaneously (sc) in the morning, Insulin Mixtard 30 18 units sc in the evening. She continues to administer simvastatin 40mg. She was due to see an ophthalmologist but missed her appointment.

Write a discharge summary for this patient. Consider which other professionals may be contacted and by whom.

Suggestions for discharge summary

Dear Dr [GP]

Mrs DM was admitted under the care of Dr [consultant] on [date] with breathlessness and fevers. She was treated with IV co-amoxiclav and oral clarithromycin for a community-acquired pneumonia. Her renal function had deteriorated as a result of poor oral intake and, as a result, we stopped her ramipril temporarily. She was also reviewed by the diabetic team who advised stopping her metformin and commencing her on insulin as her blood glucose levels were consistently high, at 20mmol/L.

We would be grateful if you could monitor her renal function and reintroduce her ramipril at a reduced dose of 2.5mg once it returns to her baseline level of creatinine [x], urea [y] and potassium [z]. Her renal functions at discharge were as follows: creatinine [a], urea [b] and potassium [c].

Since she missed her ophthalmology appointment as a result of this admission, we would be grateful if you could arrange a further outpatient appointment. Please could you also review in your diabetic clinic and refer to the diabetic team at [hospital name] if required.

Drug history

No known drug allergies

Meds on admission

Ramipril 5mg daily

Metformin 750mg twice daily

Simvastatin 40mg daily (at night)

Meds on discharge

Insulin Mixtard 30 20 units sc morning

Insulin Mixtard 30 18 units sc evening

Simvastatin 40mg daily (at night)

Ramipril: to be reviewed depending on renal function and restarted at 2.5mg

Yours sincerely

[name]

F1

Chapter summary

This chapter has provided an overview of the roles that healthcare professions have in relation to prescribing. It has highlighted the differences between independent and supplementary prescribers as well as emphasising the importance of recognising the role that non-prescribers have in assisting you in relation to your own prescribing.

The concepts of collaborative practice and interprofessional education in association with prescribing have also been described, with particular reference to the importance of effective handovers in mitigating adverse iatrogenic patient events.

GOING FURTHER

CAIPE (2002) Definition of IPE. Available online at: www.caipe.org.uk/about-us/defining-ipe

Dawson JF, Yan X and West MA (2007) Positive and negative effects of team working in healthcare: Real and pseudo-teams and their impact on safety. Birmingham: Aston University.

Department of Health (2004) *Building a Safer NHS for Patients: Making medication safer.* London: HMSO.

Department of Health (2005) *Creating a Patient-led NHS: Delivering the NHS improvement plan.* London: Department of Health.

Foundation Programme Curriculam (2012) Available online at: www.foundationprogramme.nhs.uk/FP_Curriculum_2012_WEB.FINAL.PDF

National Prescribing Centre (2012) *A Single Competency Framework for all Prescribers.* Available online at: www.npc.co.uk/improving_quality/resources/single_comp_framework.pdf

NHS: Patient Group Directions. Available online at: www.medicinesresources.nhs.uk/en/Communities/NHS/PGDs

Pothier D, Monteiro P, Mooktiar M and Shaw A (2005) Pilot study to show the loss of important data in nursing handover. *British Journal of Nursing,* 14 (20): 1090–1093.

Thistlethwaite J (2011) Collaboration and interprofessional working. In: McKimm J and Forrest K (eds) *Professional Practice for Foundation Doctors.* Exeter: Learning Matters, pp. 189–203.

chapter 5

Medicines Requiring Particular Care

Natalie Bryars

Achieving your medical degree

This chapter will help you begin to meet the following requirements of *Tomorrow's Doctors* (General Medical Council (GMC), 2009):

17. Prescribe drugs safely, effectively and economically.

    (c) Provide a safe and legal prescription.

    (e) Provide patients with appropriate information about their medicines.

    (f) Access reliable information about medicines.

It will also link to:

Good Medical Practice (GMC, 2013a)

and

Good Practice in Prescribing and Managing Medicines and Devices (GMC, 2013b), particularly paragraphs 6–11, 28, 31 and 53.

Chapter overview

After reading this chapter you should be able to:

- recognise why these medicines need particular care when they are prescribed;
- apply the national guidance concerning the prescribing of these medicines;
- prescribe these medicines safely.

Introduction

For more than 10 years, the National Patient Safety Agency (NPSA) collected information on medication errors using a national reporting and learning system. When trends were identified, they issued national recommendations to prevent recurrence (NPSA, 2007b). Healthcare organisations have had a responsibility to implement these recommendations and prevent patient harm. This has resulted in the creation of the category 'never events' (Department of Health, 2012). Organisations that have implemented safe processes should be able to prevent these errors and they should no longer happen. Refer to Chapter 7 for more information and a complete list of 'never events' involving medication.

Through the national reporting of medication errors, the NPSA identified the medicines most frequently associated with severe harm (NPSA, 2009). These include anticoagulants, injectable sedatives, opiates, insulin, antibiotics, chemotherapy agents, antipsychotics, infusion fluids, potassium chloride injection, oral methotrexate and antiplatelets. Many of these have been the focus of NPSA safety alerts and require particular care when they are prescribed.

You should be aware that the key functions and expertise for patient safety developed by the NPSA have now transferred to NHS England. This means that patient safety issues identified through the national reporting of medication errors are now managed by them rather than the NPSA. However, at the time of writing, this is a new change and no further alerts have been released. The NPSA is therefore referred to as a source of information throughout this chapter.

What's the evidence?

NPSA alerts come with supporting information. These provide the evidence for why it was necessary to release the specific safety alert. This includes information about how many incidents have been reported for each medicine, what the incidents were, what patient harm has occurred and what has contributed to the errors occurring. These can still be accessed at www.npsa.nhs.uk.

In addition, the NPSA released summary reports of all the medication-related errors reported to them over a specified time period. These reports contain trend analysis, which provides evidence of the patient safety issues of which prescribers should be aware. They also provide examples of real medication errors that have caused patient harm. The following two reports can also be accessed at the NPSA website:

National Patient Safety Agency (2007) Safety in doses. *Improving the Use of Medicines in the NHS: Learning from national reporting.*

National Patient Safety Agency (2009) Safety in doses. *Improving the Use of Medicines in the NHS: Learning from national reporting.*

Specific medicines

Oral methotrexate

Methotrexate is used to treat a number of non-cancer indications, such as rheumatoid arthritis, psoriasis and Crohn's disease. In these cases, it is prescribed as a single weekly dose. Since 2004, the NPSA has received 165 reports of patient safety incidents involving oral methotrexate (NPSA, 2006a). Dosing errors were a common cause of severe patient harm, especially when methotrexate was prescribed more frequently than once weekly. This has been so well publicised by the NPSA that the Department of Health (2012) has classed it as a 'never event'.

When prescribing oral methotrexate, you should always include the correct:

- dose;
- route;
- frequency;
- day of the week when methotrexate should be taken.

In addition, only one strength of methotrexate tablet should be used (usually 2.5mg).

When prescribing oral methotrexate on an inpatient prescription chart, you must state that it is a weekly dose and the other six days of the week should be struck out (Figure 5.1).

Methotrexate is a cytotoxic drug and every patient who takes it needs to be closely monitored. Serious patient harm can occur if the correct monitoring is not carried out (NPSA, 2006a).

What monitoring do you think needs to take place in these patients?

For all patients prescribed methotrexate, the full blood count, liver function tests and renal function tests need to be closely reviewed. Patients also need to be monitored for signs of methotrexate toxicity/intolerance, such as breathlessness, dry persistent cough, vomiting, diarrhoea, sore throat, bruising or mouth ulcers. Were you aware that there is a patient-held monitoring booklet to help with this? These are available at www.npsa.nhs.uk and should be issued to all patients taking oral methotrexate. These booklets should give details of the dose being taken and the monitoring schedule that is being followed. They should also give details about the patient's folic acid regime.

Why do you think it is important to consider folic acid for patients prescribed methotrexate?

Drug ③ METHOTREXATE		(PO)								
		SC	6							
Date 7/1/2012	Dose 10mg	IM	(8)	X	X	X	X	X		X
Additional Instructions Weekly on Monday		IV	12							
			14							
Full Signature & Bleep A. Doctor	Pharm	Supply	18							
			22							

Figure 5.1   Prescription chart for methotrexate

Methotrexate affects folate metabolism and can cause side-effects that are similar to folate deficiency. Patients who experience mucosal or gastrointestinal side-effects may benefit from folic acid. Although this is an unlicensed indication, as long as it is not taken on the same day as methotrexate, the effectiveness of methotrexate has not been shown to be reduced.

Whenever you prescribe methotrexate you should make sure you are informing patients about how to take methotrexate safely. Telling them about potential side-effects and how these should be managed can reduce the risk of patient harm. Patient information leaflets are available at www.npsa.nhs.uk to help with this and should be given to patients before treatment is started.

Anticoagulants

Anticoagulants are a class of medicines that are commonly identified as causing patient harm and hospital admissions (Pirmohamed *et al.*, 2004). When the NPSA contacted the medical and pharmacy defence organisations and the NHS Litigation Authority for available data, they were presented with 600 reported cases of patient harm from the use of anticoagulants in the UK up to the end of 2002 along with 120 reported deaths (NPSA, 2006b). Of these, 77% were related to warfarin and 23% related to heparin.

The NPSA undertook a literature review and completed a risk assessment on the use of anticoagulants in the NHS. This found that inadequate competencies of healthcare professionals prescribing and monitoring patients on anticoagulants and failure to implement professional guidelines contributed to the high incidence of patient harm. Do you have the knowledge and training needed to prescribe anticoagulants safely? E-learning packages are available to assist with the initiation and maintenance of anticoagulant therapy at www.bmj. com. If you haven't used the BMJ learning areas, they are worth logging into. Additional work competencies for anticoagulant therapy are available at www. npsa.nhs.uk.

Oral anticoagulants

Oral anticoagulants are used to treat a number of medical conditions, including atrial fibrillation, deep-vein thrombosis, pulmonary embolism, arterial thromboembolism and heart valve replacements. The oral anticoagulant most commonly prescribed in the UK at present is warfarin. Warfarin can be difficult to prescribe as dosing is specific to each individual patient. Overanticoagulation can cause patient harm through haemorrhage and underanticoagulation can cause patient harm through thrombosis, both of which can be life-threatening.

The British Society for Haematology Committee has produced clear guidance for the management of patients on warfarin (Keeling *et al.*, 2011). It has also produced recommendations on safety indicators to complement these guidelines (Baglin *et al.*, 2006).

ACTIVITY 5.1 READ THE FOLLOWING ARTICLES

Keeling D, Baglin T, Tait C, Watson H, Perry D, Baglin C, Kitchen S *et al.* (2011) Guidelines on oral anticoagulation with warfarin, fourth edition. *British Journal of Haematology*, 154 (3): 311–324. Available online at: www.b-s-h.org.uk

Baglin T, Cousins D, Keeling D, Perry D and Watson H (2006) Recommendations from the British Committee for Standards in Haematology and National Patient Safety Agency. *British Journal of Haematology*, 136: 26–29. Available online at: www.npsa.nhs.uk

What are the key learning points for you as a future prescriber of anticoagulants?

Initiating warfarin

Before you initiate a patient on warfarin, you should be clear about:

- the indication;
- the target international normalised ratio (INR);
- the duration of treatment;
- if the patient is at high risk from warfarinisation (e.g. has congestive cardiac failure, infection, interacting drugs, liver failure, diarrhoea, a raised baseline INR);
- if the patient has any contraindications;
- the loading regime (an age-related dosing algorithm should always be followed when fast loading of warfarin is required);
- if parenteral anticoagulation is required until oral anticoagulation with warfarin is established;
- if the patient is of childbearing potential (warfarin is teratogenic and should not be given in the first trimester of pregnancy. It can also increase the risk of haemorrhage and should be avoided in the last trimester of pregnancy).

You'll need to carry out or order baseline tests before warfarin therapy can be started. These include a baseline INR, liver function tests, activated partial thromboplastin time (APTT) and platelets. Are you confident about how to interpret each of these tests? Additional information can be found at www.labtestsonline.org.

You need to be confident that patients are fully able to manage their warfarin therapy, as well as being able to attend frequent INR monitoring – something especially important in patients who are frail or confused, or who have a chaotic lifestyle (Keeling *et al.*, 2011).

You must give appropriate counselling to all patients who are prescribed oral anticoagulants at the start of their therapy. The NPSA (2007) developed a patient information pack for oral anticoagulants; this can be viewed on the NPSA website. This includes:

- an information booklet, providing patients with essential information about warfarin, including potential side-effects and how they should be managed;

- a record book, where all details about the patient's dose and blood test results should be recorded;
- a card for the patient's purse or wallet, which alerts others to the fact that the patient is taking warfarin.

You must also be clear about who will be responsible for dosing and monitoring the patient. Most patients are managed by an anticoagulant service (based in hospital or the community). If you make a referral to an anticoagulant service, you need to make sure that you provide them with all the information they need to dose the patient effectively. This includes the diagnosis, the target INR, the planned duration of treatment, the dose of warfarin on referral and any current medication (Keeling *et al.*, 2011).

Monitoring warfarin

If your patient is taking an anticoagulant, he or she must have regular INR checks and appropriate warfarin dose adjustment. Warfarin interacts with a wide range of medications (see *British National Formulary* (BNF) Appendix 1), many producing an increase in anticoagulant effect. It can also be affected by changes in diet and alcohol consumption. As a prescriber, you should be aware of this and make appropriate prescribing decisions and dose adjustments. Many fatalities and permanent harm events with warfarin were associated with inadequate laboratory monitoring and clinically significant drug interactions, usually involving non-steroidal anti-inflammatories (NPSA, 2006b).

Parenteral anticoagulants

Heparin is an injectable anticoagulant. It is used in higher doses to treat venous and arterial thromboembolism, as well as in lower doses for thromboprophylaxis. It is fast-acting, so is often used until oral anticoagulation can be established, as well as at times when oral anticoagulants are deemed unsuitable.

Unfractionated heparins

Therapeutic doses of sodium and calcium heparin have to be monitored on a regular basis. This ensures that the dose being given is achieving the required level of anticoagulation and the most common way to test this is with the APTT test.

Frequent dose adjustments are usually required to ensure effective anticoagulation and to prevent complications of bleeding. Both inadequate laboratory monitoring and inappropriate dosing are frequent causes of harm to patients in secondary care (NPSA, 2006b).

Low-molecular-weight heparins (LMWH)

LMWHs are used both to treat venous and arterial thromboembolism, and for thromboprophylaxis, in the majority of hospitals within the UK. LMWHs are prescribed according to the weight of the patient for many indications and blood tests are not generally needed to ensure effective anticoagulation.

Frequent causes of patient harm include failure to weigh patients accurately, failure to identify the clinical need to initiate treatment and an inability to calculate an appropriate dose (NPSA, 2010a). The renal function of the patient also needs to be taken into consideration. LMWH is renally cleared and must be used with caution in patients with renal failure due to an increased risk of bleeding. In these patients, you may need to reduce the dose or use an unfractionated heparin. You can find further dosing information in the BNF.

ACTIVITY 5.2

Consult the BNF and familiarise yourself with the LMWHs currently licensed for use. What dose of dalteparin would you prescribe for a female patient with deep-vein thrombosis who has normal renal function and weighs 62kg?

Dalteparin 12,500 units should be prescribed once daily by subcutaneous injection for this patient.

Antimicrobials

There is evidence to suggest that antimicrobials are associated with more prescribing errors than any other class of medicine (Lewis *et al.*, 2009). Inappropriate antimicrobial prescribing in secondary care has resulted in increased costs and patient length of stay (Dunagan *et al.*, 1989). This is due to treatment failure, toxicity, delayed and omitted doses and adverse reactions.

Narrow-spectrum antibiotics are generally preferred to broad-spectrum ones. However inexperienced prescribers can tend not to use these. This increases the risk of antimicrobial resistance and healthcare-associated infections (Department of Health, 2003). Indeed, healthcare-associated infections are said to affect an estimated one in ten NHS hospital patients per year.

The Health Protection Agency (2010) has produced a guidance document for managing infections in primary care, called *Management of Infection Guidance for Primary Care for Consultation and Local Adaptation*. This is available at www. hpa.org.uk. This will help you to understand the principles of treatment with antimicrobials and how to treat common infections effectively. It also provides you with links to other relevant national guidance.

In secondary care, the Department of Health (2011a) has produced guidelines for antimicrobial stewardship called *Stay Smart Then Focus: Guidance for antimicrobial stewardship in hospitals* (available at www.dh.gov.uk). This sets out a clear pathway for the use of antimicrobials that hospitals are expected to adhere to. It also establishes clear responsibilities for all prescribers of antimicrobials. Are you aware of what these are?

As a prescriber, you should not start an antimicrobial unless there is clinical evidence of bacterial infection. Where antimicrobials are indicated, you should prescribe using the local guidelines. You should therefore make sure that you are familiar with your local antimicrobial prescribing policy. You should also know how to contact your local clinical microbiologist as he/she can provide advice on appropriate treatment options.

Wherever possible you should obtain samples prior to prescribing or administering antimicrobials and ensure that cultures and sensitivities are utilised for prescribing decisions, where available. When you prescribe antimicrobials you should document the indication, the course length or review date, the route and the dose clearly in the patient's medical records and prescription chart. Treatment should then be commenced within 1 hour of diagnosis where infection is life-threatening.

It is essential that you review the clinical diagnosis and the continuing need for antibiotics within 48 hours and make a clear plan of action. Prescribing decisions include:

- stopping the antimicrobial (the shortest duration that gives an appropriate clinical outcome should be used);
- switching the route from intravenous (IV) to oral (this should happen as soon as clinically appropriate);
- changing the antimicrobial (this should be in line with culture and sensitivity results or the clinical signs/symptoms of infection);
- continuing the antimicrobial.

You need to make sure that you document this review and any subsequent decision clearly in the patient's medical records.

You must always check the allergy status of a patient before antibiotics are prescribed. Reports of patients being prescribed and administered a drug to which they have a documented allergy remain high. This is especially true with penicillin and can be fatal.

ACTIVITY 5.3

Have a look at this list of antimicrobials. Do you know which ones contain penicillin?

- Amoxicillin
- Timentin
- Flucloxacillin
- Augmentin
- Piperacillin
- Tazocin
- Co-fluampicil

- Magnapen
- Pivmecillinam
- Penicillin v
- Benzylpenicillin
- Co-amoxiclav
- Piperacillin with tazobactam
- Ampicillin

All of the antimicrobials listed above are penicillins.

Insulin

You will know that insulin is used for the treatment of type 1 and type 2 diabetes. However, did you know that between November 2003 and November 2009, the

NPSA (2010a, b, 2011) received 16,600 reports of medication incidents involving insulin? Of these, 24% were reported as having caused patient harm. Common causes of patient harm included:

- inappropriate doses being prescribed or administered;
- the wrong type of insulin being prescribed or administered;
- inappropriate abbreviation of the term 'unit' leading to ten-times dose administration errors;
- delayed or omitted doses.

Look at chapter 6.1.1 on insulins in the BNF. You will see that there are over 20 different types of insulin available in the UK at present. They can be human insulin analogues or extracted from animals. They can be rapid-acting, short-acting, intermediate-acting or long-acting. They are available as a mixture of different insulins, known as biphasic insulins. They are also available in a number of different injection formats. Can you see the potential for confusion when prescribing or administering insulin? This is especially the case with insulins that have similar-sounding names, such as NovoRapid and NovoMix, or insulins that have small differences in their name, such as Humalog, Humalog Mix25 and Humalog Mix50.

Inappropriate dosing and wrong product selection with insulin can cause severe patient harm and patient death. This has been so well publicised by the NPSA that the Department of Health (2012) has classed it as a 'never event'.

Do you have the knowledge and training needed to prescribe insulin safely? E-learning packages are available to assist with the safe use of insulin and insulin IV infusions. These were developed by NHS Diabetes, an organisation that has since been superseded by NHS Improving Quality (NHS IQ) and can be accessed at NHS England at www.england.nhs.uk.The BNF will also provide you with essential prescribing information about each insulin. In addition, MIMS Online (http://www. mims.co.uk) will give you information about administration and the duration of action of different insulins.

ACTIVITY 5.4

Complete the e-learning package on the safe use of insulin from NHS Diabetes at www. diabetes.nhs.uk or NHS Improving Quality (NHS IQ) at www.england.nhs.uk. What are the key learning points for you as a prescriber of insulin?

To reduce prescribing errors with insulin, always write:

- insulin and type (e.g. insulin glargine);
- brand name (e.g. Lantus);
- the device to be used (e.g. Innolet);
- the dose clearly and the word 'units' in full (e.g. 10 units).

Patients should also be empowered to take an active role in their treatment with insulin. In support of this, the NPSA has developed a patient information booklet, along with a patient-held record, the insulin passport, which will document the patient's current insulin regime. This will also enable a safety check for you as the prescriber. These can be obtained at www.npsa.nhs.uk and prescribers are required to provide insulin passports when initiating or providing repeat prescriptions for insulin.

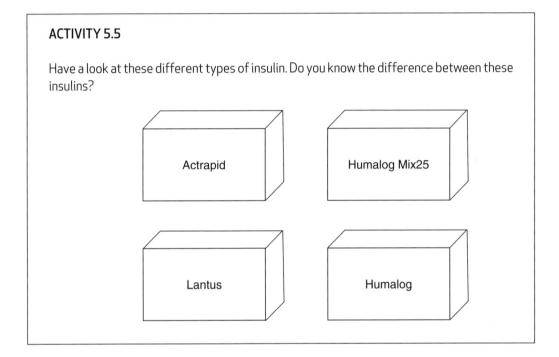

ACTIVITY 5.5

Have a look at these different types of insulin. Do you know the difference between these insulins?

Actrapid

Humalog Mix25

Lantus

Humalog

Actrapid is a short-acting insulin, usually given 15–30 minutes before meals and in diabetic emergencies.

Humalog is a rapid-acting insulin analogue, usually given with or immediately after meals.

Humalog Mix25 is a biphasic insulin. This means it is a mix of a rapid-acting and intermediate-acting insulin. It is usually given twice a day.

Lantus is a long-acting insulin, usually given once a day.

Opioids

You will know that opioids are commonly used to treat acute and chronic pain. However, are you aware how often opioids are involved in medication errors? By July 2008, the NPSA had received reports of over 4,200 dose-related patient safety incidents concerning opioids (NPSA, 2008). Patient harm commonly occurred due to inappropriate doses being prescribed or administered. This was especially true when the patient had no history of taking opioids and could be very sensitive to their effects. This has been so well publicised by the NPSA that the Department of Health (2012) has classed it as a 'never event'.

Whenever you prescribe an opioid, you must take a full patient history to determine any previous opioid use. This includes the doses, formulations and the frequencies of both regular and as-required opioids. This enables you to make sure that the dose you are prescribing is safe for the patient.

Information on starting doses, as well as dose conversions, of opiates is available in the BNF and can be found under each individual drug name, or in the 'Prescribing in palliative care' section. Additional information can also be sourced in the *Palliative Care Formulary*, in local policies and guidelines or alternatively go online to www.palliativedrugs.com.

When you increase the dose of an opioid, you should make sure that the calculated dose is safe for the patient. Dose increases should not normally be more than 30–50% higher than the previous dose.

Wrong product selection is another common cause of errors. You should therefore make sure you are familiar with all the products you are prescribing.

ACTIVITY 5.6

Do you know the difference between these products?

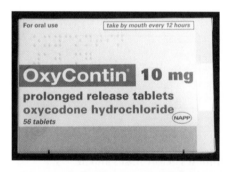
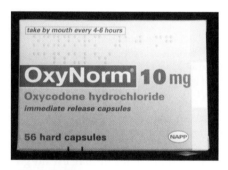
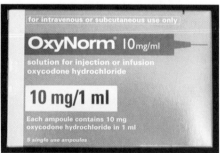
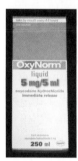

Thanks to Napp Pharmaceuticals for allowing us to photograph these medicine packets.

OxyContin is a brand of modified-release oxycodone. It should be prescribed twice daily and doses administered at 12-hour intervals.

Oxycodone is twice as potent as morphine.

OxyNorm is a brand of immediate-release oxycodone capsules or oral liquid. It is prescribed for acute pain relief and breakthrough pain.

Oxycodone injection also has the brand name OxyNorm. It is twice as potent as oral OxyNorm.

Case Study 5.1

A patient with chronic pain has been well controlled on oral morphine, taking sustained-release morphine sulphate tablets (MST) 40mg twice daily. He has compliance problems due to difficulties in swallowing tablets and a decision is made to start him on fentanyl patches.

What dose of patch would you prescribe for this patient? When would you advise him to stop taking the MST and start with the fentanyl patches? What would you prescribe him for breakthrough pain?

A fentanyl 25 microgram/hour patch is equivalent to 90mg of oral morphine in 24 hours. One patch should be applied to dry, non-hairy skin on the upper arm or torso. It should be removed every 72 hours and replaced with a new patch, sited on a different area. Evaluation of the analgesic effect should not be undertaken until the patch has been in place for at least 24 hours as it takes time to achieve steady-state concentrations. The previous analgesia should be phased out gradually, with the last dose of MST being taken at the time the first patch is applied. If the patient can swallow liquids, morphine sulphate oral solution can be prescribed for breakthrough pain. The dose is usually a sixth of the regular total daily dose, given every 4 hours if necessary. In this case, the dose would therefore be 15mg.

The Misuse of Drugs Act 2001 means that there are many legal requirements relating to the prescribing of opioid analgesics. Do you know what these are? The BNF provides guidance on prescribing for controlled drugs and drug dependence.

Potassium

IV potassium is frequently used to treat severe or symptomatic hypokalaemia. However the NPSA (2002) identified a risk to patients from errors occurring during the IV administration of potassium solutions. These are ampoules or vials of concentrated potassium chloride or potassium phosphate solution. These can be fatal if given inappropriately, causing cardiac arrest.

The Department of Health (2012) has classified the maladministration of potassium chloride solution as a 'never event'. Therefore potassium chloride or potassium phosphate ampoules should only be stocked in designated areas for use by specialist staff and ready-made potassium infusions should be used wherever possible.

When you prescribe a potassium infusion, you will need to think about the concentration of potassium and the rate of administration and ensure that these are safe for the patient. This will be dependent on how the infusion will be administered.

When potassium infusions are given via a peripheral IV cannula, the maximum concentration is usually 40mmol of potassium per litre. However, 80mmol of potassium per litre may be used in fluid-restricted patients with a large peripheral cannula. The maximum infusion rate should not usually exceed 10mmol of potassium per hour. However if the patient has continuous electrocardiogram (ECG) monitoring 20mmol of potassium per hour can be used (UCL Hospitals, 2010). The infusion should also be administered via a volumetric pump to ensure the accuracy of the administration rate.

Concentrations greater than 80mmol of potassium per litre must be given via a central line (UCL Hospitals, 2010). This is to reduce the risk of phlebitis. They must be administered via a volumetric pump and continuous ECG monitoring is required. The maximum infusion rate should not usually exceed 20mmol of potassium per hour. Faster rates may occasionally be needed but continuous ECG monitoring is required due to the risk of serious arrhythmias or cardiac arrest.

When a patient is receiving IV potassium, the serum potassium and other serum electrolytes and blood glucose should be monitored. The patient should be monitored for signs of local pain, vein irritation and extravasation, especially at higher concentrations. The patient should also be monitored for ECG changes, paraesthesia, confusion and weakness, especially at higher concentrations and faster administration rates.

For further information on IV drug administration, check out the UCL Hospitals (2010) *Injectable Medicines Administration Guide*, the Medusa Injectable Medicines Guide (available online) and local policies and procedures. In addition, did you know that you can obtain a Summary of Product Characteristics and patient information leaflet for most medicines at www.medicines.org.uk?

Oral chemotherapy

Oral anticancer medicines are commonly administered in primary and secondary care, with 24 million doses being administered during 2006–2007 (NPSA, 2008b). The NPSA received high numbers of patient safety incidents concerning oral anticancer medicines. Common causes of patient harm included:

- wrong doses being prescribed;
- wrong frequency being prescribed;
- wrong course duration being prescribed.

The standards for prescribing oral anticancer medicines should be the same as those for injectable chemotherapy (NPSA, 2008b). This means that they should only be initiated by a cancer specialist and prescribed only in the context of a written protocol or treatment plan. The patient should also be given full verbal and written confirmation about the oral cancer medication upon initiation. This must include details on the intended regime, the treatment plan and any monitoring arrangements that are in place.

As a non-cancer specialist, you may occasionally be asked to prescribe ongoing anticancer medication for a patient. You must always discuss this with a cancer specialist first to ensure it is appropriate. You must then make sure you have access to all written protocols and treatment plans, including guidance on monitoring and the management of toxicity, before you prescribe anything.

Your local cancer network can provide you with a range of chemotherapy education resources, such as competency packs, teaching packs and work books. They will also provide you with the local treatment protocols for adults and children and relevant patient information. If you do not know how to access your local cancer network team, log on to http://ncat.nhs.uk and you will be directed.

Chapter summary

In this chapter we have discussed medicines that require particular care when they are prescribed. We have considered some of the evidence showing for why this is and commonly reported errors associated with their use.

For each of these medicines, we have considered some of the national guidance on how they should be prescribed. We have also considered how to access this guidance, together with other learning resources available to you. Familiarising yourself with these will help you to develop the necessary knowledge and skills to prescribe safely.

As mentioned earlier, NPSA has transferred to NHS England and patient safety issues identified through the national reporting of medication errors are now managed by them rather than the NPSA. At the time of writing, no further alerts have been released, but check www.england.nhs.uk.

GOING FURTHER

Department of Health: www.dh.gov.uk
Health Protection Agency: www.hpa.org.uk
National Patient Safety Agency: www.npsa.nhs.uk
NHS England: www.england.nhs.uk

chapter 6

Prescribing for Specialist Patient Groups

Daniel Greer

Achieving your medical degree

This chapter will help you begin to meet the following requirements of *Tomorrow's Doctors* (General Medical Council (GMC), 2009):

8. (f) Demonstrate knowledge of drug actions: therapeutics and pharmacokinetics; drug side effects and interactions, including for multiple treatments, long-term conditions and non-prescribed medication; and also including effects on the population, such as the spread of antibiotic resistance.

17. Prescribe drugs safely, effectively and economically.

    (d) Calculate appropriate drug doses and record the outcome accurately.

    (f) Access reliable information about medicines.

It will also link to:

Good Medical Practice (GMC, 2013a)

and

Good Practice in Prescribing and Managing Medicines and Devices (GMC, 2013b), particularly paragraphs 6–11 and 53–54.

Chapter overview

This chapter will cover prescribing in the following specialist groups:

- older people;
- patients with renal impairment;
- patients with hepatic impairment;
- children;
- pregnant women;
- breastfeeding women.

You should take particular care when you are prescribing for patients in these groups as changes in pharmacokinetics and pharmacodynamics mean that the potential for adverse drug reactions and prescribing errors is higher than in other patient groups. The chapter will explain the underlying factors that affect prescribing in these groups and give advice on principles to be followed and sources of information that are best used to guide the choice of drugs and doses.

After reading this chapter you should be able to:

- describe the pharmacokinetic and pharmacodynamic changes that occur in these groups;
- identify key drug classes associated with problems in each group;
- use relevant clinical and biochemical parameters to assess the degree of renal or hepatic impairment with respect to altering drug doses;
- use appropriate methods to calculate doses in children;
- apply key principles for reducing risk when prescribing for pregnant women and breastfeeding women;
- use appropriate information sources to guide drug choice and dose in these specialist groups.

Prescribing for the older person

Older people are more likely to be on multiple medicines. People over 60 make up 20% of the population but receive 52% of all prescriptions, and in the over-75 age group 36% are taking four or more medicines (termed polypharmacy) (Department of Health, 2001). This high prevalence of medication use, together with comorbidity and changes in pharmacokinetics and pharmacodynamics, increases the risk of encountering adverse drug reactions and drug interactions when you prescribe for this patient group.

What pharmacokinetic changes take place in the older person?

Pharmacokinetics describes how the body handles medicines, and consists of four stages: absorption, distribution, metabolism and excretion. Important age-related changes occur principally with distribution, excretion and metabolism (Mangoni and Jackson, 2003).

ACTIVITY 6.1

Look up digoxin in the *British National Formulary* (BNF) – what advice is given under cautions for dosing in older people? Discuss with a colleague what this advice might mean in clinical practice.

Distribution

With increasing age the proportion of body fat increases and the proportion of body water decreases. For water-soluble drugs the smaller proportion of body water means that the same dose results in higher serum levels in older people. Examples of this include digoxin and gentamicin. As you will have seen in the BNF from the activity above, the dose of digoxin should be reduced in older people.

For fat-soluble drugs distributing into the larger proportion of body fat, the main result is a prolonged half-life, i.e. it takes longer to clear a dose from the body, with an increased risk of accumulation if doses are not adjusted. An example of this is nitrazepam. This is a long-acting benzodiazepine, and the half-life increases from approximately 30 to 40 hours in the older person, making it an inappropriate choice for night sedation, as significant drug levels are still likely to be present the following morning, which may increase the risk of falls and confusion.

Excretion

The principal organ responsible for excretion of medicines in the body is the kidney. With increasing age, renal function declines at a mean of about 1% a year, but with large variability between patients (Lindeman, 1992). Comorbidities such as heart failure and diabetes can also worsen renal function, making it important that you check renal function in older people and adjust doses accordingly. See the section on prescribing for patients with renal impairment later in this chapter for how to do this in practice.

Metabolism

Although there is an age-related decline in hepatic blood and liver volume, the large reserve of the liver means that you are unlikely to need to adjust doses of medicines metabolised in the liver unless there is evidence of liver disease. This is dealt with later in this chapter.

What pharmacodynamic changes take place in the older person?

Pharmacodynamics describes what the medicine does to the patient. In general, older people have increased sensitivity to medicines, even allowing for the changes in serum levels that may occur as a result of pharmacokinetic changes. Most commonly this is due to a decline in homeostatic reserve. Some common examples are given below.

Postural hypotension

The normal homeostatic response to maintain blood pressure on standing is tachycardia and vasoconstriction, both of which may be impaired in older people. Medicines that inhibit this response are more likely to produce postural hypotension, which may increase the risk of falls. Examples include beta-blockers (inhibition of tachycardic response) and medicines with vasodilatory side-effects (e.g. calcium channel blockers, nitrates, alpha-blockers). Medicines that are central nervous system (CNS) depressants (e.g. opiates, benzodiazepines) may also decrease sympathetic outflow and increase postural hypotension. Falls in the older person are a major cause of morbidity and mortality, and national guidance recommends that you should review medicines that may have contributed to falls as part of a wider multifactorial assessment in those who fall (NICE, 2004).

Postural sway

Postural stability is impaired in older people, and medicines that increase postural sway, such as benzodiazepines and opiates, may contribute to an increased risk of falling.

What's the evidence? Medicines and falls

A pair of meta-analyses by Leipzig *et al.* (1999a, b) have looked at the association of medicines and falls. In the first, type IA antiarrhythmic agents, digoxin and diuretics were weakly associated with falls, but not angiotensin-converting enzyme (ACE) inhibitors, calcium-channel blockers, beta-blockers, centrally acting antihypertensive agents, nitrates or analgesics. The second study found a small but consistent association between the use of psychotropic medicines and falls. This included antipsychotics, hypnotics, antidepressants and benzodiazepines.

A Cochrane meta-analysis (Gillespie *et al.*, 2009) looking at randomised controlled trials for interventions to reduce falls found that withdrawal of psychotropic medication decreased the rate, but not the risk, of falls (relative risk 0.34, 95% confidence interval 0.16–0.73).

Routine withdrawal of cardiac medicines to prevent falls in older people is not recommended, though they should be reviewed in the presence of symptomatic postural hypotension.

As the evidence linking psychotropic medicines with falls is stronger, national guidance recommends that *older people on psychotropic medications should have their medication reviewed, with specialist input if appropriate, and discontinued if possible to reduce their risk of falling* (NICE, 2004, p. 10).

Cognitive function

Medicines that act on the CNS may worsen cognitive function, particularly where there is pre-existing cognitive impairment. Examples include antidepressants, antipsychotics, benzodiazepines and opiates. Cholinergic transmission is considered to play an important role in cognitive function, with the result that medicines with anticholinergic side-effects (e.g. oxybutynin, hyoscine and amitriptyline) may lead to confusion in older people. When older people present with acute confusion or delirium you should always review their medicines for potential causative agents.

Visceral muscle function

Constipation is more common in older people, and drug therapy is often one of the contributing factors. Anticholinergics, opiates and tricyclic antidepressants may worsen constipation and you should review these if possible before further medicines are added to treat the constipation. Urinary retention may be a problem in older males with benign prostatic hypertrophy: medicines with anticholinergic side-effects may contribute to this as they reduce smooth-muscle contraction in the bladder. Conversely, bladder instability with symptoms of urge incontinence is more common in older people, and use of diuretics may worsen this problem. When you prescribe loop diuretics (e.g. furosemide) you should discuss with your patient to take doses no later than 2p.m., otherwise diuresis is likely to continue after bedtime.

Renal function

As discussed above, renal function declines with age. As well as the effect this has on the excretion of medicines, declining renal function will mean there is less homeostatic reserve. You should monitor renal function closely if you need to prescribe medicines that may further reduce renal function, particularly when used in combination with each other. Examples include diuretics, ACE inhibitors, non-steroidal anti-inflammatory drugs (NSAIDs) and gentamicin.

What other high-risk medicines are there in older people?

From the examples described above, you can see that the two most important classes of medicines that require you to be cautious when prescribing in the older person are medicines that act on the CNS, and medicines acting on the cardiovascular system. There are some other classes of medicines that also require careful use in older people.

ACTIVITY 6.2

Look for a warfarin prescription chart or guidelines in your hospital. What is the suggested regime for loading in older people? If you were considering starting warfarin for an older person, what patient factors might influence whether you think this medicine would be safe to use in your patient?

Warfarin

Older people are more sensitive to warfarin and require lower doses. Most warfarin loading guidelines suggest a lower loading dose of 5mg for older patients (rather than 10mg). Safe use of warfarin requires regular blood tests for international normalised ratio (INR) and subsequent dose adjustment. If patients have cognitive impairment, you should consider whether there is sufficient support in place from carers to allow this process to take place safely.

Non-steroidal anti-inflammatory drugs

Gastrointestinal bleeding is the most important adverse effect of NSAIDs, and older people are more at risk of this adverse effect. Compared to people aged 25–49 years, people aged 60–69 had 2.4 times the risk of a serious gastrointestinal complication, while those aged 70–80 were found to have 4.5 times the risk (Hernandez-Diaz and Rodriquez, 2000). Current guidance suggests that you should always prescribe a gastroprotective agent with an NSAID, normally a proton pump inhibitor (e.g. lansoprazole or omeprazole). NSAIDs can also reduce renal function and worsen cardiac failure.

Hypoglycaemic medicines

In older people with diabetes, hypoglycaemia can lead to significant morbidity and even mortality. Long-acting sulphonylureas such as glibenclamide are more likely to cause hypoglycaemia and should be avoided; shorter-acting agents such as gliclazide are preferred.

Other risk factors for medicine-related problems in older people

ACTIVITY 6.3

What other factors can you think of that might be likely to lead to medicine-related problems in older people? Discuss your responses with a colleague to see if you have come up with similar ideas.

Aside from use of high-risk medicines, other factors have been identified as important factors associated with medicines-related problems in older people (Department of Health, 2001).

Taking four or more medicines

Polypharmacy increases the risk of drug interactions and adverse drug reactions.

Recent discharge from hospital

This is a high-risk period as changes to medicines have frequently been made, both intentional and unintentional. Good communication between primary and secondary care is essential. This should include what medicines have been started and stopped, reasons for these changes and instructions for any ongoing monitoring.

Physical factors

Poor vision and hearing can affect the ability of patients to receive and use information about how to take medicines correctly. Patient information leaflets that come with dispensed medicines are often in a small font size. Larger-print leaflets are available from www.xpil.medicines.org.uk.

Physical dexterity will affect the ability to take medicines (e.g. opening blister packs and tablet bottles, using inhalers). You may need to liaise with the pharmacy with regard to assessing patients and providing alternatives.

Mental state

Confusion, disorientation and depression are all risk factors for medicines-related problems.

Lack of social support

Many older people will have formal or informal carers who can help with medicines, and this can help to overcome some of the risks identified above. When older people are not taking their medicines independently you should ensure that carers are informed about new medicines and medication changes. Where this support is absent problems are more likely to arise, and you may need to work with the multidisciplinary team to provide extra support with medicines.

Prescribing for patients with renal impairment

In patients with renal impairment, the two most important factors that you need to consider are whether the drug is renally excreted and whether the drug is renally toxic. This is because the consequences of toxicity are likely to be more serious when there is less homeostatic reserve, as discussed earlier in this chapter.

Dose adjustment in renal impairment

The degree of dose adjustment required in renal impairment will depend on the proportion of the drug that is eliminated by renal excretion and the dose-related toxicity. Dose reduction can be achieved by either reducing the dose itself or extending the dosing interval. If an immediate effect is required, a loading dose may be required as the increased half-life means that time to steady-state levels will be increased.

How can you estimate renal function?

In order to adjust doses of drug eliminated by the renal route, you need to be able to quantify the degree of renal impairment. The two most common methods in use

are the Cockcroft and Gault equation and the modification of diet in renal disease
(MDRD) equation.

Creatinine clearance – Cockcroft and Gault equation

The relatively constant rate of production of creatinine in individual patients
together with almost exclusive glomerular filtration means that creatinine clearance
(CrCl) should reflect glomerular filtration rate (GFR). The Cockcroft and Gault
formula (Box 6.1) is the most well-established formula for estimating creatinine
clearance.

Box 6.1 Cockcroft and Gault formula

$$CrCl\,(mL/min) = \frac{(140 - age) \times weight\,(kg) \times F}{Creatinine\,(micromol/L)}$$

where F = 1.04 female, 1.23 male. Use ideal body weight if the patient is obese.

MDRD equation

In line with the *National Service Framework for Renal Services* (Department of
Health, 2005), the MDRD equation is recommended as the standard method of
estimating GFR. This provides an estimation of renal function per 1.73m², i.e. an
average body surface area.

Scenario 6.1

Mrs DS, an 85-year-old woman, has chronic kidney disease. She presents with dehydra-
tion, fever and loin pain. She also has unilateral swelling of the left calf. A provisional diagnosis of pyelonephritis and probable deep-vein thrombosis is made. Intravenous fluids
are started, and the registrar asks you to start piperacillin-tazobactam and treatment
dose enoxaparin.

Her urea and creatinine are 15mmol/L and 150micromol/L. Estimated GFR is found to
be 30mL/min/1.73m² . She weighs 50kg. You notice her urea and creatinine are normally
around 8mmol/L and 110micromol/L.

What dose of piperacillin-tazobactam and enoxaparin should she be given? Use the BNF
and relevant Summary of Product Characteristics (SPC) (www.medicines.org.uk) to find
the appropriate dose.

Although the estimated GFR is ready to hand, this woman weighs only 50kg, and therefore absolute GFR or CrCl using the Cockcroft and Gault equation should be used. There is no height available so body surface area cannot be calculated, hence CrCl is easier to use.

Using the Cockcroft and Gault equation, this works out at 19mL/min.

For piperacillin-tazobactam, the BNF advises a reduced dosing frequency dosing of 4.5g every 12 hours for CrCl <20mL/min. As the calculated CrCl is only just below the threshold of 20mL/min, you should use clinical judgement and be prepared to increase the frequency to every 8 hours if the patient does not respond to antibiotic therapy.

The BNF for enoxaparin refers to the product literature, where the SPC advises a reduced dose of 1mg/kg daily where CrCl is below 30mL/min; therefore you should prescribe 50mg once daily.

You should monitor renal function closely, as it is likely to improve with rehydration. Should this patient's renal function return to baseline (creatinine 110micromol/L), this equates to a CrCl of 26mL/min, and the piperacillin-tazobactam dose should be increased to 4.5g every 8 hours.

Prescribing for patients with liver disease

Prescribing for patients with liver disease can be challenging. Unlike in renal disease, there is no direct measure that allows you to quantify liver function in terms of ability to metabolise drugs. Variation in the type (e.g. acute versus chronic, cholestatic versus hepatitis versus cirrhotic) and severity of liver disease will affect how drug metabolism is altered. This makes it difficult to make definitive dosage recommendations.

How would you adjust doses in liver disease?

The most important indicators of a reduced metabolic function are a raised INR and a reduced albumin. If this is the case you may need to reduce the dose of liver-metabolised drugs.

Sometimes medicines may have been studied in patients with liver disease and there are specific recommendations in the BNF or SPCs (available at www.medicines.org.uk). These are most commonly based on the Child–Pugh category of liver disease, and were developed to predict mortality rather than as an indicator of metabolic function.

Where the drug has not been studied in liver disease, it is possible to make a number of recommendations based on the pharmacokinetics of the drug and likely changes that will occur in liver disease, though this is often difficult to predict. Your local medicines information centre will be able to help with advice as interpreting information is often not straightforward.

Drug choice with regard to complications of liver disease

If you have a patient with liver failure under your care, you are likely to encounter some of the complications of liver disease, such as encephalopathy, variceal bleeding and ascites. You may need to adjust drug therapy if these are present.

Encephalopathy

Generation of ammonia by bacteria in the large bowel is thought to contribute to encephalopathy, hence agents that cause constipation should be used with caution or given with laxatives. Examples include opiates, tricyclic antidepressants, 5HT3 antagonists, antidiarrhoeals and antimuscarinic drugs (e.g. procyclidine, oxybutynin, antispasmodics).

Drugs that affect the CNS should also be used with caution or avoided, as their sedating effects may increase the risk of, or worsen, encephalopathy. Examples include opiates, tricyclic antidepressants, benzodiazepines, sedating antihistamines and antipsychotics.

Bleeding

Coagulopathy is a complication of liver disease, and hypersplenism secondary to portal hypertension may also result in thrombocytopenia. Variceal bleeding may also occur. Therefore any drug that increases the risk of bleeding should be used with caution or avoided in patients with these complications. Examples include NSAIDs, antiplatelets, anticoagulants, and selective serotonin reuptake inhibitors (e.g. fluoxetine).

Ascites

A high sodium intake may worsen ascites. You should avoid using sodium chloride 0.9% as a diluent for intravenous drugs if compatibility allows, and avoid soluble/effervescent preparations as they are often high in sodium content.

Case Study 6.1: Choice of antiemetic in liver disease

A patient with a history of alcoholic liver disease presents with encephalopathy. His liver function tests are as follows:

Alkaline phosphatase	183	(70–300IU/L)
Bilirubin	133	(3–15 micromol/L)
Alanine aminotransferase	25	(0–35IU/L)
Albumin	24	(37–49g/L)
INR	2.9	

The patient complains of nausea. Which of the following antiemetics is the most appropriate choice?

Cyclizine, metoclopramide, prochlorperazine, ondansetron, domperidone

---

As the INR is raised and the albumin is low, your patient is likely to have reduced metabolic capacity. He also has encephalopathy, therefore you should avoid agents that might worsen this.

Cyclizine and prochlorperazine should be avoided as they may be sedating and could worsen encephalopathy. Metoclopramide can have CNS effects and should also be avoided. Ondansetron could potentially be used, but can cause constipation, which could worsen encephalopathy. The BNF advises a maximum of 8mg daily in moderate to severe impairment.

Despite the BNF recommendation to avoid, domperidone is likely to be the antiemetic of choice. Despite being extensively metabolised by the liver, it has few adverse effects, and does not cross the blood–brain barrier, so will not worsen the encephalopathy. In view of the impairment in metabolic function, the starting dose should be reduced (e.g. 50%) and titrated up to 10mg three times daily (North-Lewis, 2008).

Can you use potentially hepatotoxic drugs in liver disease?

With the exception of sodium valproate and methotrexate, hepatotoxicity is no more likely to occur in someone with pre-existing liver disease; however the consequences are likely to be more serious. You may need to make a clinical judgement as to whether to prescribe.

You should consider whether a less hepatotoxic drug can be used to treat the same problem, or whether treatment can be delayed until liver function improves. If neither is possible you will need to balance the risks of liver toxicity (based on the reported probability and severity) versus the benefits of the drug therapy you wish to use. You may wish to discuss this with a more senior member of your team.

Prescribing for paediatric patients

Children differ from adults in their response to drugs. Choice of dose is very important as there are huge variations in weight across the age range from birth to 18 years, and also large changes in physical development, which affect drug distribution, excretion and metabolism. The most dramatic changes occur in the first year of life.

What pharmacokinetic changes occur in children?

Absorption

Up to about 6 months of age gastric emptying time is longer than in adults. Overall bioavailability (the proportion of a dose reaching the circulation) generally remains the same, but rate of absorption is slower and therefore onset of action may be delayed in neonates.

Increased topical absorption may be seen in neonates and infants, due to the stratum corneum being thinner. As the body surface area to weight ratio is higher in this age group, there is a greater potential for adverse effects.

You should generally avoid giving intramuscular injections in paediatric patients. The lack of muscle mass means that injection is very painful, and the variability in blood flow means that absorption into the systemic circulation can be unpredictable.

Distribution

Important changes in body fat/water composition occur in the first year. Fat content rises from 12% to 30% from term to 1 year, while body water drops from 75% to 60%. For water-soluble drugs (e.g. gentamicin), larger doses on an mg/kg basis are required in a neonate compared to an older child in order to achieve therapeutic levels.

Metabolism

The liver is not fully developed until 6–12 months of age, hence drug metabolism is generally reduced in neonates. From years 1–5, however, metabolic activity is increased compared to adults, and larger doses of metabolically cleared drugs (e.g. theophylline) may be required compared to adults on an mg/kg basis.

ACTIVITY 6.4

Look up the dose of chloramphenicol in the *BNF for Children* (BNF-C: Paediatric Formulary Committee, 2013). How does the dosing regimen compare for:

- a neonate up to 14 days;
- a neonate between 14 and 28 days;
- a child > 28 days old.

What are the risks of chloramphenicol toxicity in a newborn?

Grey-baby syndrome is a rare side-effect that can occur following intravenous use of chloramphenicol in neonates (Pharmacia Ltd, 2009). It is due to accumulation of toxic chloramphenicol metabolites secondary to impaired glucuronidation in neonates. The dosing frequency is therefore much less in younger neonates.

Excretion

Renal function in neonates is less than adults, matures by 1 year of age and is then better than adults before declining. The dosing of renally excreted drugs reflects this; for example, the recommended frequency of dosing of gentamicin increases with age from 2.5mg/kg every 24 hours in a neonate less than 29 weeks' postmenstrual age, up to 2.5mg/kg every 8 hours in a 1-month-old (Paediatric Formulary Committee, 2013).

Sources of information on dosing

You should obtain doses of medicines from a paediatric dosage handbook. In the UK, although the adult BNF contains some paediatric doses, the recommended gold standard source is the BNF-C (Paediatric Formulary Committee, 2013).

How do you calculate doses in paediatrics?

There are three main methods that you will come across when calculating doses for children: body weight, body surface area and dosing by age.

Body weight

This is the most common method to calculate doses. In the BNF-C this is stated as mg/kg. It is good practice to document body weight on prescriptions to allow doses to be double-checked by nursing or pharmacy staff.

Generally the calculated dose should not exceed the maximum recommended dose for an adult. For obese children you may need to use ideal body weight. Doses are usually expressed in terms of a single dose together with the recommended frequency (e.g. 1mg/kg twice daily). Occasionally doses are quoted as total daily dose (e.g. 3mg/kg daily in three divided doses). You should check this carefully, as confusing the total daily dose with the single dose could result in an overdose.

Body surface area

Many physiological parameters relevant to drug handling correspond better with body surface area. This can be calculated from weight and height using nomograms, but this can be difficult to obtain in acutely unwell children. For this reason relatively few drugs are dosed in this way, e.g. cytotoxics. A table of body surface area according to body weight is available at the back of the BNF-C.

Dosing by age

Some drugs with a wide therapeutic range are quoted as a single dose for an age range (e.g. for amoxicillin 1 month–1 year 62.5mg three times daily, 1–5 years 125mg three times daily). This simplifies dosing regimens; however you should take care if children are underweight for their age as this could result in an overdose. Tables of mean weight by age are available at the back of the BNF-C.

Whatever method is used to calculate the dose, make sure that the dose can be practically measured. The standard oral syringe is supplied when liquid medicines are prescribed in doses other than multiples of 5mL, and is marked in 0.5mL divisions.

ACTIVITY 6.5

A 54kg child of 12 years requires prophylactic trimethoprim 2mg/kg at night for recurrent urinary tract infections. Use the BNF-C to calculate an appropriate dose.

2mg/kg = 108mg. However the maximum dose is 100mg.

Trimethoprim suspension is 50mg/5mL and 100mg tablets are available. A dose of 100mg should be prescribed, which will be easy to measure using a 5mL spoon or by tablet.

ACTIVITY 6.6

A 5-year-old child weighing 20kg requires intravenous aciclovir for herpes zoster infection. The child's height is not readily available. Use the BNF-C to calculate an appropriate dose.

Using the tables in the BNF-C, a 20kg child has a body surface area of $0.79m^2$. A dose of $250mg/m^2$ every 8 hours is recommended = 197.5mg. For practical purposes this should be rounded to 200mg every 8 hours.

Excipients

Where possible use sugar-free preparations, particularly for long-term medication. The BNF-C states which branded preparations are sugar-free. Rarely, some liquid preparations have a high level of alcohol (e.g. some preparations of phenobarbital elixir), which is unsuitable for children. Benzyl alcohol, which is a preservative used in some injectable products, should be avoided in neonates as it has been associated with a fatal syndrome (gasping syndrome) in preterm neonates. Information on these excipients is also indicated in the BNF-C.

Unlicensed medicine use

Many medicines are only licensed for use in adults, as the manufacturer will have only investigated their safety and efficacy in adults, either due to commercial reasons or difficulty in recruiting children into clinical trials. Almost three-quarters of medicine use on neonatal wards, and about one-quarter of medicines on paediatric wards, is prescribed outside of their licence (Department of Health, 2004).

Prescribing unlicensed medicines or medicines outside of their licence increases your professional responsibility and potential liability. You should ensure that such prescribing is done on an informed basis, and all licensed alternatives have been exhausted.

ACTIVITY 6.7

A 5-year-old child requires an antihistamine for travel sickness. Using the BNF-C to guide you, what are the most appropriate choices?

Dosing information for a 5-year-old is available for cinnarizine, cyclizine and promethazine in the BNF-C. However cyclizine is unlicensed in children under 6 years, while cinnarizine and promethazine are licensed. You should choose one of these in preference.

Prescribing in pregnancy

Drugs can have harmful effects on the embryo and fetus at any stage, yet for some patients denying medication of benefit may lead to uncontrolled disease which may be more harmful to both the patient and fetus than the risk of continuing therapy. If you are asked to prescribe for a pregnant woman, you will therefore need to make a careful assessment of the risks and benefits to both the patient and fetus. You will also need to consider this if prescribing in women of childbearing age if there is a potential for pregnancy.

Teratogenic effects of drugs

The strict definition of a teratogen is one that causes congenital malformations; however the definition in practice normally includes any agent that causes structural, functional or behavioural abnormalities to the fetus.

Assessing the teratogenic risks of medicines is difficult. Ethical issues prevent the inclusion of pregnant patients in randomised controlled trials, hence most of the data in humans come from epidemiological studies and case reports. The incidence of major congenital malformations in the general population is 2–3%; of these, only 1–2% are thought to be drug-related (UKMi, 2012). This means that to show a statistically significant association large studies are required of the order of tens of thousands of patients. For this reason no drug can be considered safe beyond all doubt, but older drugs tend to be used in preference as there will have been more experience with these. Animal studies can be useful in identifying likely teratogens, but extrapolation to humans cannot be assumed.

Warfarin

Warfarin is teratogenic and should not be given in the first trimester. There is a risk of placental, fetal or neonatal haemorrhage, especially during the last few weeks of pregnancy and at delivery. If pregnant women require anticoagulation, low-molecular-weight heparins are normally used.

ACE inhibitors

Avoid in pregnancy unless essential. They may adversely affect fetal and neonatal blood pressure control and renal function; skull defects and oligohydramnios have also been reported. See section 2.5 of the BNF for an overview of managing hypertension in pregnancy.

Isotretinoin

Avoid, as it is teratogenic. Effective contraception must be used. You may have noticed that more details are given in the BNF on the timing and methods of contraception advised for women of childbearing potential.

Amoxicillin

Amoxicillin is not known to be harmful.

What factors affect teratogenicity?

There are a number of general principles that affect teratogenicity that can be useful for you to consider when considering potential risk.

Timing of exposure

Extensive damage during the pre-embryonic phase (conception to 17 days) is thought to result in failure to implant and miscarriage, while minor damage will be repaired by division of undifferentiated cells, with subsequent normal development. You will need to take care if there is uncertainty around dates, or if the drug has a long half-life.

The embryonic phase (days 18–55) is the highest-risk period for exposure and damage during this period is most likely to result in malformations.

During the fetal period (56 days to birth), organs continue to develop and some remain susceptible to damage, such as the cerebral cortex and kidney. Functional abnormalities (e.g. deafness) may also occur.

Use in the final trimester may result in pharmacological effects to the neonate, for example, bradycardia with atenolol, respiratory depression with opiates. Long-term exposure of the fetus to maternal drug therapy may also lead to withdrawal symptoms after birth. Examples of this include benzodiazepines, opiates and antidepressants (Shaefer *et al.*, 2007).

Dose

Teratogenic effects are generally dose-dependent; hence there is a general recommendation that you should prescribe the lowest effective dose in pregnancy.

Multiple drug therapy

Risk of teratogenicity may be increased if the number of drugs taken concomitantly is increased.

Maternal pharmacokinetic changes

Significant changes in drug distribution may occur because of an increase of up to 50% in blood volume, and a mean increase of 8 litres in body water. Kidney function also changes, with an increase in glomerular filtration rate of 50%, which may affect drugs that are excreted predominantly by the kidneys. You may need to carry out more frequent monitoring for drugs with narrow therapeutic indices (e.g. carbamazepine, phenytoin, lithium, digoxin) (Anderson, 2005; Pavek *et al.*, 2009).

What are the key principles for reducing risk in pregnancy?

- Assess risk–benefit – the risk of exposure of the fetus must be balanced against the risk of uncontrolled disease if therapy is stopped.
- Consider non-drug treatments where possible and only prescribe drugs if essential.
- If possible, avoid all drug use during the first trimester.
- Avoid new drugs – there is usually little information available on their safety in pregnancy.

- Avoid multiple drug therapy.
- Avoid known teratogens in women of childbearing age. If this is not possible, the potential risks should be discussed with the patient.
- Use the lowest effective dose for as short a period as possible.
- Consider the need for therapeutic drug monitoring and dose alteration for drugs with narrow therapeutic index.

Sources of information

The BNF gives brief information on use in pregnancy under individual drug monographs. The SPC may give more information, but will tend to err on the side of caution for medicolegal reasons. You can obtain detailed information from the UK Teratology Information Service by phone on 0844 892 0909, and online through TOXBASE (www.toxbase.org).

Case Study 6.2: Balancing the risks and benefits of drugs in pregnancy

Mrs C is a 25-year-old woman with a history of ulcerative colitis. She has had two admissions to hospital with severe flares, and was started on azathioprine 6 months ago. This has maintained her in good remission and she has been free of flares since.

She is now wishing to start a family, and is concerned about the safety of azathioprine, as the patient information leaflet states not to take it if you are pregnant or you think you might become pregnant.

On consulting the BNF, it advises that there have been reports of premature birth and low birth weight following exposure to azathioprine, particularly in combination with corticosteroids, and that spontaneous abortion has been reported. The information from TOXBASE on azathioprine concludes that: *the available data do not currently indicate an overall increased risk of adverse pregnancy outcome following azathioprine use in pregnancy.*

You discuss this with Mrs C, and also explain the difficulties of extrapolating risk caused by azathioprine from that caused by inflammatory bowel disease. You also discuss the benefits of remaining on azathioprine with regard to maintaining disease remission. You discuss how fertility in active disease is reduced, that active disease in itself is a risk factor for premature birth and low birth weight, and that surgery if necessary for uncontrolled disease may also reduce fertility (Mowat *et al.*, 2011).

Following this discussion of the risk and benefits, you offer your opinion that on balance the best course of action might be for Mrs C to continue her azathioprine while trying for a family, and during any eventual pregnancy. She agrees with this.

Prescribing in breastfeeding

Breastfeeding mothers who require prescribed medicines are likely to be concerned about the effects of drugs on their child, hence it is important that you understand the principles of use. This is to ensure that infants are protected from adverse drug reactions from maternal medication, and equally that both necessary maternal medication and breastfeeding can continue wherever possible, as breastfeeding is widely acknowledged as the best form of nutrition for infants (WHO/UNICEF, 2003). Most drugs pass in to breast milk to some degree, though the overall dose that the infant receives is normally low and normally below a therapeutic level for the infant.

What factors affect infant risk?

There are a number of factors which affect the risk of an infant being exposed to drugs from breast milk.

Milk-to-plasma ratio

This is the ratio of concentration of a drug in breast milk compared to maternal plasma levels. Drugs pass into milk to a varying degree, governed by various physicochemical properties. Low ionisation, low molecular weight, high lipid solubility and low protein binding all lead to greater passage into the milk. Most medicines however have a milk/plasma ratio of less than 1.

Maternal plasma levels

A low milk/plasma ratio does not necessarily suggest that a medicine is safe. More important is the maternal plasma level, as if plasma levels of the drug are low, then the level in breast milk will also be low.

Bioavailability

Some medicines are poorly absorbed, or are metabolised to a large degree by the infant before reaching the systemic circulation (the first-pass effect). If this is the case, it is unlikely there will be significant effects even if there is drug present in the breast milk.

Infant maturity

As discussed in the section on paediatrics, neonates and premature infants will not have fully developed kidney and liver function needed for elimination of drugs, and therefore are more at risk of accumulating drugs ingested via breast milk. Drugs that have long half-lives and active metabolites may compound this problem.

Adverse drug reaction profile

The side-effects of the drug are the main factor when you are assessing risk. Of particular concern are cytotoxic drugs, radionuclides and iodine-containing drugs. Combination therapy with drugs with similar side-effects will also be of concern as these effects may be additive, for example, antipsychotic therapy and antiepileptics.

What general principles should I follow?

As with use in pregnancy, there are some general principles you should follow to try and minimise exposure to the infant:

- Avoid unnecessary maternal use – in particular, avoid complementary and alternative medication because of a lack of data, and advise mothers to seek advice before purchasing any over-the-counter products.
- Assess risk–benefit in individual cases – consider particular risk factors such as infant prematurity and multiple maternal medicines. Consult specialist information sources if necessary (see below).
- Minimise exposure – use the lowest effective dose for the shortest possible time.
- Consider local therapy (e.g. topical/inhaled) which normally results in lower maternal plasma levels and therefore lower passage into milk.
- If the drug has a short half-life, advise taking the dose immediately after feeding to avoid feeding at peak milk concentrations.
- Avoid drugs with toxic side-effects in adults or children (e.g. cytotoxics).
- Avoid new drugs – older drugs are more likely to have data to guide use in breastfeeding.
- Monitor the infant for adverse effects.

Sources of information

As for use in pregnancy, the BNF gives brief information on use in breast milk under individual drug monographs. The SPC for a drug will again tend to err on the side of caution. Your local medicines information service will be able to give you more detailed advice where BNF advice is not definitive.

Chapter summary

This chapter has dealt with prescribing in the following specialist groups:

- Older people: pharmacokinetic and pharmacodynamic changes were outlined. Examples of high-risk medicines were given, highlighting in particular medicines acting on the cardiovascular system and CNS. Other factors associated with medicines-related problems in older people were discussed.
- Patients with renal impairment: methods of calculating renal function were discussed, followed by using appropriate reference sources to adjust drug doses.

- Patients in liver impairment: the key pharmacokinetic changes in liver disease were outlined, followed by how the complications of liver disease affect drug choice.
- Children: pharmacokinetic differences to adults were highlighted. The different methods of calculating appropriate doses were compared, and principles of unlicensed medicine use in the group were discussed.
- Prescribing in pregnancy and breastfeeding: key factors affecting teratogenic risk and risk to the breastfeeding infant were covered, followed by principles for reducing risk.

For each group key information sources guiding appropriate drug choice and dose have been highlighted.

GOING FURTHER

Ashley C and Currie A (2008) *The Renal Drug Handbook*, 3rd edn. Abingdon: Radcliffe Medical.
The principal resource beyond the British National Formulary for advising on drug dosing in renal impairment.

Department of Health (2004) *National Service Framework for Children, Young People and Maternity Services: Medicines for children and young people.* London: Department of Health. Available online at: www.dh.gov.uk/prod_consum_dh/groups/dh_digitalassets/@dh/@en/documents/digitalasset/dh_4090563.pdf
This national document sets out the standards for medicines use in children.

Meador K, Reynolds MW, Crean S, Fahrbach K and Probst C (2008) Pregnancy outcomes in women with epilepsy: A systematic review and meta-analysis of published pregnancy registries and cohorts. *Epilepsy Research*, 81 (1): 1–13.

National Prescribing Centre (2000) Prescribing for the older person. *MeReC Bulletin* (online), 11 (10): 37–40. Available online at: www.npc.nhs.uk/merec/other_non_clinical/resources/merec_bulletin_vol11_no10.pdf
This is a good overview of the principles of prescribing in older people.

North-Lewis P (2008) *Drugs and the Liver*. London: Pharmaceutical Press.
A detailed textbook on the principles of drug use in liver impairment.

TOXBASE: www.toxbase.org
This website holds pregnancy summaries on maternal exposures to various drugs and chemicals, and also some data on breastfeeding. Access to TOXBASE is free to NHS and NHS-affiliated departments, units and practices in the UK.

chapter 7

Common Errors

David Alldred

Achieving your medical degree

This chapter will help you begin to meet the following requirements of *Tomorrow's Doctors* (General Medical Council (GMC), 2009):

8. (f) Demonstrate knowledge of drug actions: therapeutics and pharmacokinetics; drug side effects and interactions, including for multiple treatments, long-term conditions and non-prescribed medication; and also including effects on the population, such as the spread of antibiotic resistance.

Outcomes 2 – The doctor as a practitioner

17. Prescribe drugs safely, effectively and economically.

   (a) Establish an accurate drug history, covering both prescribed and other medication.

   (e) Provide patients with appropriate information about their medicines.

   (f) Access reliable information about medicines.

   (g) Detect and report adverse drug reactions.

   (h) Demonstrate awareness that many patients use complementary and alternative therapies, and awareness of the existence and range of these therapies, why patients use them, and how this might affect other types of treatment that patients are receiving.

It will also link to:

Good Medical Practice (GMC, 2013a)

and

Good Practice in Prescribing and Managing Medicines and Devices (GMC, 2013b), particularly paragraphs 8–11 and 44, 45.

Chapter overview

Accurate and error-free prescribing is fundamental to ensuring patients benefit from their medicines and do not suffer harm. In this chapter, the prevalence and nature of prescribing errors will be explored along with the causes of prescribing errors. Solutions to minimising the risk of erroneous prescribing will be discussed.

After reading this chapter you will be able to:

- define prescribing errors and understand the prevalence and nature of prescribing errors;
- explain the consequences of prescribing errors with particular reference to high-risk medicines;
- discuss the causes of prescribing errors;
- reduce the risk of you making a prescribing error.

What are prescribing errors and how often do they occur?

Medication errors have been defined as *a failure in the treatment process that leads to, or has the potential to lead to, harm to the patient* (Ferner and Aronson, 2006). They can occur in the prescribing, dispensing, administration or monitoring of medicines (Alldred *et al.*, 2008). In this chapter, we will focus on your role as a prescriber and therefore only prescribing errors will be considered. Dean *et al.* (2000) defined 'clinically meaningful' prescribing errors as occurring when:

> as a result of a prescribing decision or prescription writing process, there is an unintentional significant (i) reduction in the probability of treatment being timely and effective; or (ii) increase in the risk of harm when compared with generally accepted practice.

It is difficult to compare studies of prescribing error prevalence due to different definitions and methods of data collection (Franklin *et al.*, 2005). What is clear, however, is that prescribing errors are common in all settings. A systematic review of the prevalence of prescribing errors in hospitals found a median error rate of 7% (interquartile range 2–14%) of all medication orders (Lewis *et al.*, 2009). A study of prescribing errors made by first-year foundation trainee doctors in UK hospitals found a mean error rate of 8.4% (Dornan *et al.*, 2009). In UK general practice, Shah *et al.* (2001) found an error rate of 7.5% and a study in care homes for older people found an error rate of 8.3% (Barber *et al.*, 2009).

ACTIVITY 7.1

How many reports of medication incidents do you think are received by the National Patient Safety Agency (NPSA) in a year? If you are working in a group, see what the others think. Remember that this is reports processed, so the actual number may be significantly higher.

In 2007, the NPSA received over 80,000 reports of medication incidents and this was the third largest group of incidents reported (NPSA, 2009).

Think about the type of errors that may be included here.

There are many types of prescribing error, with dosage errors being the most common (Lewis *et al.*, 2009). Other types of error include: incomplete prescriptions, omission of medicines, illegible prescriptions, dose frequency errors, incorrect formulation, drug–disease interactions, drug–drug interactions, prescribing unnecessary medicines and errors in transcription (Alldred *et al.*, 2008; Lewis *et al.*, 2009). Not all of these are the responsibility of the prescriber, but many are.

What are the consequences of prescribing errors?

Fortunately, the majority of errors do not result in significant harm to patients: 96% of the medication incidents reported to the NPSA were judged to be of no or low harm (NPSA, 2009). However, 100 incidents led to serious harm or death, with 32% being attributable to prescribing error. In addition to serious harm, as with adverse drug reactions (see Chapter 8), errors also have the potential to reduce quality of life and can result in patients not benefiting fully from evidence-based therapy. Errors may lead to patients losing confidence in their doctor and the healthcare system. It should also be borne in mind that errors can have a significant impact on the healthcare professionals who commit them.

ACTIVITY 7.2

Considering the other chapters in this book, particularly Chapter 8, what types of medicines do you think are most likely to be involved in error? Discuss this with colleagues and see if you agree.

In the secondary care setting, antimicrobials are most commonly involved in errors, followed by cardiovascular medicines, central nervous system medicines, fluids/electrolytes/parenteral nutrition and gastrointestinal medicines (Lewis *et al.*, 2009). From the data reported to the NPSA, the medicines most frequently associated with severe harm include anticoagulants, injectable sedatives, opiates, insulin, antibiotics (allergy-related), chemotherapy, antipsychotics, infusion fluids, potassium chloride injection, oral methotrexate and antiplatelets (NPSA, 2007a, 2009; Patient Safety First, 2008). Sixty-two per cent of incidents that were fatal or caused severe harm involved injectable medicines, with 71% of incidents leading to death or serious harm being due to unclear/wrong dose or frequency, wrong medicine and omitted/delayed medicines (NPSA, 2009).

'Never events'

The Department of Health publishes a list of 'never events', which are defined as *serious, largely preventable patient safety incidents that should not occur if the available preventative measures have been implemented by healthcare providers* (Department of Health, 2011b, 2012). Several of these relate to medicines, as follows:

- wrongly prepared high-risk injectable medication;
- maladministration of potassium-containing solutions;
- wrong route of administration of chemotherapy;
- wrong route of administration of oral/enteral treatment;
- intravenous administration of epidural medication;
- maladministration of insulin;
- overdose of midazolam during conscious sedation;
- opioid overdose of an opioid-naïve patient (i.e. a patient who has never previously received an opioid);
- inappropriate administration of daily oral methotrexate.

What do you think of this list and is it useful?

Which patients are most at risk from error?

As we have seen in other chapters, as well as specific drug groups, certain types of patient may be more susceptible if errors occur. Those who are at the extremes of age (i.e. neonates, infants and older people) are at a greater risk from prescribing errors due to altered pharmacokinetics and pharmacodynamics. Patients who have multiple comorbidities and those who receive multiple medicines (polypharmacy) are also at greater risk (NPC, 2010). One of the most risky times is when patients undergo transitions in care, for example on admission to, or discharge from, hospital, or admission to a care home (Royal Pharmaceutical Society, 2011). Patients may also be at risk if they do not understand the purpose of their medicines or have difficulty taking them.

Looking ahead to the chapters on adverse drug reactions (Chapter 8) and drug interactions (Chapter 9), you will see a pattern emerging which should increase your awareness when prescribing these drugs and for these patients. Chapter 6 has also examined these ideas.

Why do prescribing errors happen?

As Seneca (1–65 CE) noted 2,000 years ago, to err is human. The psychology of human error has been studied in critical safety industries (e.g. nuclear, aeronautics) and is now widely applied in medicine to understand the causes of errors in order to develop solutions to minimise their prevalence and impact (Vincent, 2010). Key to human error theory is a recognition that the systems in which you as doctors work can contribute to error (Dean *et al.*, 2002). For a prescribing act to be successful, two conditions need to be fulfilled: (1) an appropriate plan needs to be formulated;

and (2) the plan needs to be successfully executed (Aronson, 2009; McDowell *et al.*, 2009). If the plan is wrong, then a mistake occurs. A failure to execute an appropriate plan is termed a slip or lapse.

Mistakes will happen; there are very few, if any, practitioners who have not made an error at least once. Your task is to ensure this happens rarely. You need to learn from errors and ensure that, if they were preventable, the lesson is clearly learned.

Mistakes

Knowledge-based mistakes result from a lack of knowledge about a patient or drug. Examples include prescribing penicillin without finding out whether a patient had previously suffered an anaphylactic reaction to penicillin, or prescribing Augmentin to a penicillin-allergic patient without realising that it contains a penicillin (Aronson, 2009). Mistakes can also occur by applying bad rules or by not applying/ misapplying good rules – for example, prescribing asthma therapy for a patient with chronic obstructive pulmonary disease (Vincent, 2010), prescribing medicines for symptoms that may be the result of an adverse drug reaction and continuing to prescribe repeat medicines after the condition has been cured.

Slips and lapses

Slips and lapses are errors in executing plans (skill-based errors). Slips are errors of commission, such as selecting bisocodyl instead of bisoprolol from a drop-down computer list, whereas lapses are errors of omission, such as intending to write up a statin for a patient who has had a myocardial infarction but forgetting to do so.

Violations

Violations are intended deviations from protocol or policies (McDowell *et al.*, 2009) and include abbreviating drug names, not providing full information on the prescription and using abbreviations for dose units (e.g. µ or mcg for micrograms). Violations are usually employed to save time; however, they increase the risk of error and should be avoided.

Accident causation model

Reason (1990) developed the accident causation model to explain the causes of error. In the model, mistakes, slips/lapses and violations are described as active failures.

ACTIVITY 7.3

Think of how these active failures could occur in the place in which you practise. Discuss the ideas with colleagues and write them down.

As mentioned previously, the system in which you prescribe can contribute to error and this is influenced by organisational decisions that are termed latent conditions.

ACTIVITY 7.4

Think of examples of latent failures that you have seen in the place in which you practise. Discuss the ideas with colleagues and write them down.

An example of a latent condition would be poor systems for communicating medication histories between the GP and hospital. In addition to latent conditions, error-producing conditions also contribute to active failures and these include being tired, stressed or hungry. Error-producing conditions may also be related to the particular task at hand, or they may be related to the patient – for example, if a patient has severe dementia, which makes taking an accurate history impossible.

Ultimately, latent and error-producing conditions can result in active failures – that is to say, in prescribing errors. To mitigate against this, defences are built into healthcare systems to detect and prevent errors from reaching patients. These are discussed in the next section.

What's the evidence? Prescribing errors

A systematic review of the causes of prescribing errors in secondary care found that knowledge-based mistakes (lack of knowledge about the patient or the drug) were deemed to be the most frequent active failures (Tully et al., 2009). Slips and lapses were also found to be common. Error-producing conditions included a lack of doctor training or experience, tiredness, stress, high workload and poor communication between healthcare professionals. A reluctance to question senior doctors and inadequate training were considered to be latent conditions. The causes of errors were multifactorial, often with multiple error-producing conditions and active errors combining to lead to error.

What can be done to reduce errors?

Prescribing errors often have complex and multifactorial causes. Consequently, multifaceted solutions are required to reduce errors. Clinical governance teams are responsible for designing and implementing safer systems in the NHS; however, in this section we will focus on what you, the individual doctor, can do to reduce the risk of error.

Do you know who manages clinical governance in your organisation? Now is a good time to find out and identify their role. This will of course vary from organisation to organisation so there is no specific answer.

Reducing knowledge-based mistakes

ACTIVITY 7.5

As the prescriber, how would you attempt to reduce knowledge-based mistakes in the light of what you have just read? Discuss this with colleagues to see how they approach the potential problem. Do you agree or are you each bringing different ideas which can supplement each other?

Some of your responses should have included the following.

Knowing your patient

Having comprehensive, accurate and up-to-date information about the patient is fundamental to safe prescribing. This includes knowing the patient's conditions, drug sensitivities (allergies and previous adverse drug reactions), medication history and renal and hepatic function. Having this knowledge means that you can avoid prescribing contraindicated medicines, or you can tailor your prescribing to the individual, for example, reducing doses in renal impairment. Obtaining an accurate medication history and ensuring patients are prescribed the correct medicines is particularly important when patients are transferred to and from different settings. This process is called medicines reconciliation and the National Institute for Health and Clinical Excellence (NICE: recently renamed National Institute for Health and Care Excellence) has produced guidelines on how and when medicines reconciliation should be carried out (NICE, 2007).

Knowing your drugs

Clearly, to be able to prescribe safely you need a good working knowledge of drugs, including their indications, dosage, contraindications, cautions, drug–drug interactions and side-effects. Given that there are thousands of medicines available to the prescriber, this is not an easy task. It is essential that you have access to high-quality information on medicines so that you can quickly obtain the information you need if you have any doubts. As well as textbooks and online materials, colleagues such as senior doctors, nurses and pharmacists will be able to give guidance. Don't be shy to ask (see Chapter 4).

ACTIVITY 7.6

Download and read *10 Top Tips for GPs* at: http://www.npc.co.uk/evidence/top_10_tips/top_10_tips_for_GPs.php

The following paragraphs relate to this document.

Avoiding slips and lapses

Avoiding slips and lapses is difficult, as by their nature, you do not know you have committed them. The risk increases when error-producing conditions such as fatigue, stress and a high workload are present. Being vigilant when you know you are tired, stressed or overworked and double-checking your prescribing (preferably with another healthcare professional) can help you to avoid them. It is especially important to double-check your prescribing when dealing with high-risk medicines (e.g. anticoagulants, insulins, opiates, chemotherapy), intravenous preparations and when completing drug calculations. Interruptions can lead to slips and lapses; if possible, try to find a quiet place to work on complex prescribing tasks and ask not to be interrupted. If you are interrupted, be vigilant for slips and lapses when you return to your task.

ACTIVITY 7.7

Complete the drug calculations found in Appendix 1 at the end of this book. You can check your answers there too once you have completed the task.

Care also needs to be taken with 'look-alike' and 'sound-alike' medicines, especially those for which the doses are similar, e.g. amiloride and amlodipine, clomiphene and clonidine; familiarising yourselves with these can help (Derby Hospitals Foundation Trust, 2012; see also Chapter 5).

Avoiding violations

It is crucial that your prescribing is legible and unambiguous to ensure safe prescribing so that the right patient receives the right medication at the right dose at the right time and by the right route. In primary care, the legibility of prescriptions has been improved by the introduction of computer prescribing. However, occasions do arise where handwritten prescriptions are still necessary in the community. In secondary care, electronic prescribing has been introduced in many hospitals for discharge prescriptions, but drug charts are usually handwritten. Common violations include not completing the prescription with sufficient detail for safe dispensing and administration, not documenting allergies, abbreviating drug names and abbreviating dosage units. It can be tempting when you have a high workload to take such short cuts; however the consequences can be catastrophic.

Build good relationships with your colleagues

One of the main defences in detecting errors is other healthcare professionals, particularly pharmacists and nurses. However, there is a tendency for junior doctors to rely on pharmacists and nurses to identify errors (Dornan *et al.*, 2009) and this complacency can potentially lead to serious events.

Speak with your patients

Your patients and their relatives/carers are often the experts on their medicines and are the last line of defence in detecting errors. Educating patients about their medicines and asking them about side-effects and any concerns that they have can lead to the identification of errors.

Regularly review medicines

Conducting regular medication reviews and ongoing monitoring of treatment is important to ensure that the continued prescription is still appropriate. You may find that your patients receive medication reviews from pharmacists and nurses in the community. You as a prescriber can refer patients for such reviews.

Utilise guidelines for safe prescribing

Your own workplace may have developed specific guidelines for the process of writing prescriptions and for making good choices about medication. Box 7.1 gives one example.

Box 7.1 Harrogate and District NHS Foundation Trust – top 10 tips for prescribing

1. Ensure correct patient's details on the prescription – full name, date of birth, unit number and address.

2. Allergies – document sensitivities or NKDA (no known drug allergies) in the relevant section of the prescription/chart.

3. Clarity – ensure prescription is legible, in black ink, capital letters, generic name (except if the *British National Formulary* (BNF) recommends brand names be used or a combination drug is prescribed where there is no generic name).

---

4. Do not use abbreviations – e.g. ISMN, FeSO$_4$ – write out in full.

5. Write out units, micrograms and nanograms in full.

6. Avoid decimal points where possible – if unavoidable, a zero should be written in front of the decimal point, e.g. 0.5mL not .5mL. Take special care with controlled drugs.

7. Rewrite dose changes – increases or decreases.

8. Cross-reference additional charts in use – on the front of the prescription chart in the 'specialist charts in concurrent use' section and as an item inside the chart if a drug is prescribed, e.g. 'warfarin – see anticoagulant chart'. If more than one prescription chart is required, circle the number of charts in use section on the front of the pre-scription chart. Ensure all drug charts are bound together.

9. As-required (PRN) medicines – must have indication, dose interval and maximum daily dose specified.

10. Contact details – is the prescriber identifiable? Are their contact details clear?

Ensure that you are familiar with the medicine and the normal dose range for everything that is prescribed.

Be clear, do not guess.

Case Study 7.1

Mr T is receiving Uniphyllin Continus (modified-release theophylline) 400mg twice daily and has developed an acute exacerbation of chronic obstructive pulmonary disease. Ciprofloxacin 500mg twice daily was pre-scribed by the GP.

- What could be the potential consequence of this?
- What type of active failure is this?
- How could this have been prevented?

Answer

Ciprofloxacin increases the plasma concentration of theophylline (you can find this in the BNF) and this can lead to theophylline toxicity. For example, Mr T could develop a supraventricular arrhythmia and convulsions.

The active failure is a knowledge-based mistake.

This could have been prevented by knowing your drug interactions or by developing the habit of checking for drug interactions in a source such as the BNF whenever a new drug is added into an existing drug regime (see Chapter 9). The dose of theophylline could have been reduced or an alternative non-interacting antibiotic prescribed.

Case Study 7.2

Mrs C was diagnosed with incontinence by Dr P who was at the end of a busy shift. He intended to prescribe the antimuscarinic oxybutynin 5mg twice daily but, in error, prescribed oxycodone 5mg twice daily.

- What could be the potential consequence of this?
- What type of active failure is this?
- How could this have been prevented?

Answer

Mrs C's incontinence would not be treated and she may suffer side-effects such as sedation, nausea and constipation from the oxycodone – an opioid.

This is a slip and probably occurred because the medicines sound similar and are used in the same dose.

This could potentially have been prevented by having an awareness of the risk of errors when tired and busy, leading to double-checking by Dr P or by a second check, for example by the pharmacist.

Case Study 7.3

Mrs A, a patient with type 1 diabetes, was admitted to hospital with acute coronary syndrome. Prior to admission, she was receiving Novomix 30 8 units in the morning and 20 units in the evening. On admission to the cardiology ward, the FY2 doctor prescribed Novomix 30 8u in the morning, 20u in the evening

- What could be the potential consequence of this?
- What type of active failure is this?
- How could this have been prevented?

The nurse could have interpreted the morning dose as 80 units, which would result in severe hypoglycaemia.

This is a violation failure.

This could have been prevented by following guidelines for safe prescribing and not abbreviating units to u. The valuable role of patients in preventing errors can also be seen here – when regular medications are being administered in hospital, patients may be the first to notice differences and so we should ensure that they are encouraged to speak up if they have any concerns.

Chapter summary

In this chapter we discussed prescribing errors, what they are and how frequently they occur. We showed that they were common in all healthcare settings and had the potential for causing serious harm to patients. We concluded that the causes of prescribing errors are multifactorial and that multiple solutions were needed to avoid or reduce their incidence. We looked at mistakes, slips and lapses and considered some ways to avoid them. Prescribing legibly and unambiguously was shown to be fundamental to assuring safe prescribing. Remember you work in a team and it is important to use the expertise of others if it helps the safe prescribing of medicines to patients.

GOING FURTHER

British Journal of Clinical Pharmacology 2009; 67 (6).
>   *This is a themed issue of the journal focusing on medication errors.*
Howard RL, Avery AJ, Slavenburg S, Royal S, Pipe G, Lucassen P and Pirmohamed M
>   (2007) Which drugs cause preventable admissions to hospital? A systematic review. *British Journal of Clinical Pharmacology*, 63: 136–147.
National Prescribing Centre: www.npc.nhs.uk/improving_safety
>   *This website supports prescribers in improving safety and managing the risk of prescribing and has many useful e-learning resources.*
NHS England: http://www.england.nhs.uk/ourwork/patientsafety
>   *The aim of NHS England is to improve health outcomes for people in England.*
NHS Patient Safety: http://www.nrls.npsa.nhs.uk
>   *This website has practical information, tools and support to improve patient safety in the NHS.*
NICE Medicines and Prescribing Support: http://www.nice.org.uk/mpc
>   *The National Prescribing Centre was integrated into NICE in 2011 and now provides advice and support for delivering quality, safety and efficiency in the use of medicines.*
Vincent C (2010) *Patient Safety.* Singapore: Wiley-Blackwell.
>   *This text reviews the evidence of risks and harms to patients and provides practical guidance on implementing safer practice.*

chapter 8

Adverse Drug Reactions

Barry Strickland-Hodge

Chapter overview

Adverse drug events (ADEs), adverse drug reactions (ADRs) and side-effects have a major impact on patients – not only on their recovery time and general wellbeing, but also on the confidence they have in your ability to prescribe safely. Some ADRs can be predicted but others are more subtle and affect only some people.

Before reading further into this chapter, find the section in the *British National Formulary* (BNF) or in the electronic BNF (www.bnf.org) that discusses ADRs. It is usually near the beginning of the book; for example, in BNF 65 it starts on page 12. In particular, look at the section called side-effects in the BNF and consider what the BNF includes and what is not included. You will see that the BNF describes what you should do if you suspect an ADR and how to report it.

After reading this chapter you will be able to:

- describe what is meant by ADEs, ADRs and side-effects;
- discuss the incidence and effect of ADRs;
- describe the classification and severity of ADRs;
- discuss the types of drug associated with most ADRs;
- identify the patient groups most likely to suffer from ADRs;
- apply strategies to try and avoid ADRs;
- report ADRs;
- recognise where to go for further information.

ACTIVITY 8.1 WHY SHOULD YOU, AS A DOCTOR, BE INTERESTED IN ADVERSE DRUG REACTIONS?

Think about why you as a doctor should be concerned with ADRs. Why are we concentrating on ADRs in this chapter?

Write down your answer and discuss it with a colleague.

Look again at your answer when you have finished working through this chapter, and see if your ideas have changed.

You might have said any or all of the following.
ADRs:

- cause hospital admissions;
- are the most common cause of iatrogenic injury in hospital patients;
- complicate existing disease;
- delay the cure of disease;
- mimic other diseases and may, therefore, lead to further treatments;
- result in inappropriate treatment if the drug-induced problem is not recognised;
- can affect the patient's quality of life;
- can cause patients to lose confidence in the prescriber and their treatment;
- cost the NHS over £1 billion per year.

What are adverse drug events, adverse drug reactions and side-effects?

The broadest of these terms is ADE, which covers not only ADRs but any errors from prescribing or administering drugs (see Chapter 7 for more details). The original World Health Organization definition (1970) of an ADR as opposed to

ADE *is a response to a drug which is noxious and unintended and which occurs at doses normally used for prophylaxis, diagnosis or therapy of disease.* A more recent definition is:

> *An appreciably harmful or unpleasant reaction, resulting from an intervention related to the use of a medicinal product, which predicts hazard from future administration and warrants prevention or specific treatment, or alteration of the dosage regimen, or withdrawal of the product.*

(Edwards and Aronson, 2000, p. 1255)

A side-effect of a medicine might be defined as any result that occurs in addition to the intended effect. Some side-effects can be useful. A side-effect of the antihistamine diphenhydramine hydrochloride is drowsiness; so if you have a rash that itches and you take the medication at night, it may help you sleep through the itch and help prevent you scratching. If, however, you take the same antihistamine for itch in the daytime and drive into a tree, the drowsiness was an unintended side-effect that proved noxious at the correct dose. ADRs, therefore, are always adverse, while side-effects might be useful. ADRs aren't the same as overdoses because, looking at the definition again, ADRs occur at normal doses. An overdose could be covered by the term ADE.

How often do adverse drug reactions lead to hospital admission?

Research into the frequency of ADRs that lead to hospital admission varies depending on the study design and how the term ADR is defined. Data from meta-analyses and systematic reviews suggest that the rate of admissions directly due to ADRs is 5% (Einarson *et al.*, 1993; Edwards and Aronson, 2000; Wiffen *et al.*, 2002). A large prospective observational study in Merseyside found 6.5% of admissions were due to ADRs (Pirmohamed *et al.*, 2004). It is much more difficult to estimate the level of ADRs in the community as reporting is not as efficient and trials are more difficult to conduct, but they are important and do cause problems to patients.

What's the evidence? ADRs

In the Merseyside study mentioned earlier (Pirmohamed *et al.*, 2004), the researchers found that, of 18,820 hospital admissions, 1,225 or 6.5% were due to ADRs. In 80% of these the admission was due directly to the ADR, with the most common reaction being gastric bleeding due to aspirin and non-aspirin non-steroidal anti-inflammatory drugs (NSAIDs). There were 28 deaths, again mainly due to gastric bleeding, but renal failure and lithium toxicity due to co-administration with NSAIDs were also implicated. The study was conducted in NHS hospitals in Merseyside. The conclusion was that there was an additional cost to the NHS of the ADRs which led to considerable morbidity and mortality. It is accepted that NSAIDs and other drugs which can cause ADRs have a place in therapy but prescribers need to be cautious when using them in order to reduce the burden ADRs can have on the NHS and on patients.

Most ADRs identified in the research were predictable from known pharmacology of the drugs and many represented known interactions.

What are your thoughts at this point?

There were a number of comments about the paper, with the majority being very positive. Other studies confirmed the findings, but one or two authors thought that the blame could not be put solely on doctors. Patients buy aspirin and NSAIDs such as ibuprofen at the supermarket or pharmacy and this was not highlighted in the study. Similarly, the dose of aspirin was not included in the results. Overall, monitoring, gastric protection and caution with reactive drugs and susceptible patients are essential.

How are adverse drug reactions classified?

Firstly, as with drug interactions (see Chapter 9), there are two main types of ADR: pharmacokinetic and pharmacodynamic. These relate to the ways the body acts on the drug (pharmacokinetics) and the ways the drug acts on the body (pharmacodynamics).

Pharmacokinetic ADRs

In pharmacokinetic ADRs, any problem the patient may have with drug absorption, distribution, metabolism or excretion may cause an adverse effect of a drug at normal doses in that patient. The two main pharmacokinetic factors that will potentially lead to ADRs relate to the main sites of metabolism and excretion, the liver and kidneys.

Pharmacodynamic ADRs

In pharmacodynamic ADRs, the site at which a drug acts is responsible for the resulting adverse effect. Metoclopramide and domperidone act as dopamine receptor antagonists, but only metoclopramide crosses the blood–brain barrier and hence has its action in the central nervous system as well as peripherally. In a patient with Parkinson's disease, we should choose domperidone to avoid antagonising the limited remaining dopamine in the patient's central nervous system.

Type A and type B adverse drug reactions

ADRs are divided into two main groups: type A and type B (Rawlins and Thompson, 1977).

Type A

Type A ADRs are relatively common and are often discovered during the clinical trials phase of drug development. They are usually related to the pharmacological activity of the drug and occur at normal doses in normal people. They can manifest as additive effects to the original drug effect, hence their other name, 'augmented' ADRs. They are largely predictable so warning of their possibility can be given to patients, with guidance as to what to do if they occur. They can cause high levels of morbidity but mortality is low. Examples of type A ADRs might be constipation with opioids due to their action on the gut, and dry mouth and blurred vision with tricyclic antidepressants because of their antimuscarinic effects.

Type B

Type B ADRs, on the other hand, are not predictable, which leads to their other defining name of 'bizarre'. When the reason for the ADR is found to be genetic, the ADR is often called a pharmacogenetic reaction. Type B ADRs include allergic reactions or genetic responses. Examples include rashes with penicillins.

You can read about different ADRs in Anne Lee's 2006 book, which is listed in the 'Going Further' section at the end of this chapter.

Types C–E

It has since been considered necessary by some to subdivide ADRs further into types C–E. In type C (chronic), the adverse effect develops after continuous or chronic use, such as osteoporosis after long-term steroid use. An example of type D or delayed ADRs was the use of diethylstilboestrol in pregnant mothers to prevent premature labour. In this case, teenage daughters born to these mothers were shown to develop vaginal adenocarcinoma significantly more often than other girls in the same age group. Type E or end-of-use reactions might include rebound effects after long-term use of, for example, nasal decongestants.

As a doctor, it is important to remember that you can't always predict how an individual will react to a new drug so it is important to consider carefully those drug types (see Chapter 5) and specific patient groups (see Chapter 6) which are more susceptible to reactions.

European classification of adverse drug reactions

European legislation has brought in a simple classification according to incidence of reported ADRs. This terminology is used in the Summary of Product Characteristics (SPC) for drugs, as shown on www.medicines.org.uk. These SPCs have all the legally required information about drugs marketed by companies within the Association of the British Pharmaceutical Industry, which covers the majority of those drugs you will use. The European classification is presented as percentage probabilities of developing an ADR and is shown in Table 8.1.

Table 8.1 European classification of adverse drug reactions according to incidence

Very common	More than 10%	(>1 in 10)
Common	1–10%	(1 in 100 to 1 in 10)
Uncommon	0.1–1%	(1 in 1,000 to 1 in 100)
Rare	0.01–0.1%	(1 in 10,000 to 1 in 1,000)
Very rare	Less than 0.01%	(< 1 in 10,000)

ACTIVITY 8.2 INCIDENCE OF ADVERSE DRUG REACTIONS

Look up the drug varenicline, a drug to aid smoking cessation. Look at the SPC, then look under the section called *Undesirable Effects*. Identify the cardiac adverse effects atrial fibrillation and palpitations. These are classified as uncommon. Will that make you confident in the use of the drug? Uncommon is 1 in 100 up to 1 in 1,000.

Now consider how many people smoke (say 20% (Cancer Research UK Smoking Statistics) of the adult population of, say, 50 million) and how many could be offered varenicline. How many of these could potentially be affected by atrial fibrillation or palpitations?

It seems a very broad classification. To calculate, 20% of 50 million is 10 million. If, let's say, 10% are offered varenicline, that's 1 million and if 1 in 1,000 suffer the ADR, that's still 1,000 people. The benefits of stopping smoking must not be underestimated and may in your opinion (and mine) outweigh the possible ADR but caution is required, particularly in susceptible people.

There is no correct answer to this activity and this drug was selected at random. It's your reflection, and an understanding of these classifications that matter, and will enable you to apply the same principles to other drugs too.

Serious and severe adverse drug reactions

There are two more definitions that are important, particularly when considering reporting a suspected ADR: serious and severe.

- Serious ADRs are defined as those that prove fatal; are life-threatening; are disabling or incapacitating; result in or prolong hospitalisation; produce congenital abnormalities or are considered medically significant.

- Severe ADRs may not be life-threatening or disabling but for the individual patient may be extreme. An example could be a headache, which would not normally be considered serious but may be very severe.

As a prescriber, you must report all potential ADRs for new drugs which are being monitored by the Medicines and Healthcare Products Regulatory Agency (MHRA). These are indicated by an inverted black triangle next to the drug's name in the BNF. For example, in the BNF 65, varenicline has an inverted black triangle for the brand Champix. Note that these will change depending on the edition of the BNF as they remain only while the MHRA is monitoring the particular drug. For drugs without a black triangle, only serious or severe reactions need reporting.

Which patient groups are most at risk of suffering an adverse drug reaction?

If you can identify which groups of patients are more likely to suffer an ADR then you can begin to prevent them. Age, gender, racial groups and metabolic disorders have all been cited as important factors in identifying susceptible individuals. Similarly, those on more than one medicine or who have comorbidities are also considered as being at a higher risk of ADRs. Chapter 6 goes into more detail but briefly the main points are:

- Monitor renal function in the very old and very young, particularly neonates.
- Anyone with existing renal or hepatic dysfunction will handle drugs differently.
- Women appear to be more susceptible to ADRs but the exact reason is not fully understood.
- Pregnancy, conception and breastfeeding need careful consideration.
- Some ethnic groups may be more susceptible to ADRs than others (McDowell *et al.*, 2006).
- The incidence of drug interactions and ADRs increases with the number of drugs taken.

Which drugs potentially cause more adverse drug reactions?

There are over 900 million prescription items issued in England alone each year. With such a large number of prescription medicines being taken by patients, the potential for ADRs is high. Other drugs and drug groups have been discussed further in Chapter 5.

ACTIVITY 8.3 COMMON DRUGS CAUSING ADVERSE DRUG REACTIONS

Which common drugs or drug groups do you think are most likely to cause ADRs, particularly in the community?

Discuss your answers with a colleague – have you listed the same ones?

In general, remembering that most prescribing goes on in general practice, the drug groups that are cited as having the most ADRs are:

- NSAIDs;
- anticoagulants;
- antibiotics;
- digoxin;
- diuretics;
- hypoglycaemic agents.

You may have included some of these groups but also drugs that you personally find problematic. For example, if you work in oncology you are likely to have included anticancer drugs.

Confusing new symptoms with adverse drug reactions

In an Audit Office report in 1994 called *A Prescription for Improvement*, it was suggested that some prescriptions were written to treat new symptoms which could be ADRs to a previous drug given to the patient. While treating troublesome symptoms is important, as we shall see later, ADRs should form part of your differential diagnosis. It may be that there is no choice but to treat these new symptoms but of course you may be able to stop the first drug or at least change it to one that is less likely to cause the problem.

For example, a patient is started on a 7-day course of erythromycin for an upper respiratory tract infection and experiences intense nausea from the second day. The options for treatment are:

- reassurance that nausea is common and there are only 5 more days of treatment;
- change to clarithromycin (less incidence of nausea and vomiting, same spectrum, increased cost) or another class of antibiotic;
- start antiemetic (ensure short course, not on repeat); this may be necessary if it is the only option for treatment.

The pros and cons of options – which may be different for different patients (Table 8.2) – should be discussed. For example, if you (as a patient) are frail, how concerned might you be about nausea?

Table 8.2 Examples of symptoms in a diagnosis that could be caused by drugs

Symptoms	Examples of drugs that could induce these symptoms
Dyspepsia	NSAIDs, corticosteroids
Extrapyramidal side-effects	Antipsychotics, metoclopramide
Diarrhoea	Laxatives, iron preparations, antibiotics, cytotoxics

Nausea and vomiting	Digoxin, erythromycin, iron salts
Rash or allergy	Antibiotics, allopurinol, lithium
Oedema	Calcium-channel blockers, NSAIDs
Constipation	Opioid analgesics, antihistamines, clozapine
Hypokalaemia	Diuretics
Cough	ACE inhibitors
Pseudomembranous colitis	Cephalosporin antibiotics

NSAIDs, non-steroidal anti-inflammatory drugs; ACE, angiotensin-converting enzyme.

Case Study 8.1: Confusing adverse drug reactions with new diseases

A 60-year-old man came to the surgery suffering from abdominal pain. After investigations, you were able to diagnose acute pancreatitis as (in addition to his pain) his lipase level was more than three times the upper limit. You perform the usual investigations and find the pancreatitis is not due to gallstones, duct obstruction, pancreatic cancer, autoimmune causes or alcohol. You then tested for metabolic changes (e.g. hypercalcaemia or hypertriglyceridaemia) but the tests are all negative.

The next thing to consider is: what medication is the patient taking?

If you consider that a drug treatment he is taking is responsible then discontinue the drug if possible; if not, substitute with a different medicine.

If the symptoms resolve after stopping, then drug-induced pancreatitis is probable. Inform the patient and consider re-exposure only if the benefits outweigh the risk. If the symptoms reappear on re-exposure then this is probably drug-induced pancreatitis. Stop the drug causing the symptom/condition and notify the MHRA via the Yellow Card Scheme.

What should this make you think?

Consider an ADR as part of any differential diagnosis.

This case is adapted from Nitsche *et al.* (2010).

Answer to Case Study 8.1

Some of the drugs with a definite association to pancreatitis, as reported in case reports and cited as Table 3 in Nitsche *et al.* (2010), are listed here:

Paracetamol

Azathioprine

Cimetidine

Cisplatin

Cytarabine

Didanosine

Enalapril

Erythromycin

Oestrogens

Furosemide

Hydrochlorothiazide

Interferon-α2b

Lamivudine

Mercaptopurine

Mesalamine/olsalazine

Methyldopa

Metronidazole

Octreotide

Opiates

Oxyphenbutazone

Pentamidine

Pentavalent antimonials

Phenformin

Simvastatin

Steroids

Sulfasalazine

Sulfmethaxazole/trimethoprim

Sulindac

Tetracycline

Valproic acid

Case Study 8.2: A suspected adverse drug reaction

A male patient aged 59 presents with recurrent mouth ulcers and stomach discomfort. You discuss diet and changes in dental hygiene and find no specific reason why the mouth ulcers have developed. The patient is allergic to aspirin.

His current medication history is: clopidogrel 75mg, atorvastatin 10mg, metoprolol 100mg, nicorandil 30mg.

You ask about over-the-counter medicines, which many patients use. He assures you that he takes nothing, though he has bought gels for the mouth ulcers.

Could this be related to the drugs he is taking? What about the stomach discomfort?

Answer to Case Study 8.2

Nicorandil has been associated with both mouth ulceration and gastric ulcers. In the download drug analysis prints or DAPs on the MHRA website (see section on looking at adverse drug reaction reports, below) there were 700 reports of gastrointestinal ADRs for nicorandil from a total of 2,033 reports for the period 1994–2011. Six patients died. There is no mention of mouth ulcers; however, the MHRA *Drug Safety Update* of June 2008 did suggest that both mouth ulcers and gastric ulcers were possible ADRs to nicorandil.

The SPC states that, while nausea and vomiting are common with nicorandil, gastrointestinal ulcerations such as stomatitis, mouth ulcers, tongue ulcers, intestinal and anal ulcers are rare. Remember that rare in the EU classification is 1:1,000 to 1:10,000.

As the BNF also says that mouth ulcers and gastric ulcers are potential ADRs to nicorandil, you should be aware of this.

What might your action be in this case?

In the SPC, it goes on to say that these gastric ulcers, if advanced, may develop into perforation, fistula or abscess formation. Also there is a warning that they are refractory to treatment and most only respond to withdrawal of nicorandil treatment. If ulcerations develop, nicorandil should be discontinued. Reducing the dose may help in some cases.

Therefore the appropriate action is to stop the nicorandil temporarily and check if symptoms clear. The reaction occurs rarely, appears to be dose-related and the time to ulcer onset may be days, weeks or months after starting nicorandil. Treatment should be reconsidered while investigating the ulcers further. However, in the meantime, appropriate alternative antianginals should be used (e.g. nitrates, calcium-channel blockers). The MHRA states:

> GPs and other healthcare professionals should consider nicorandil treatment as a possible cause in patients who present with symptoms of gastrointestinal ulceration. Ulcers that result from nicorandil are refractory to treatment; they respond only to withdrawal of nicorandil. Nicorandil withdrawal should take place only under the supervision of a cardiologist.
>
> (MHRA, 2008)

Adverse drug reactions and differential diagnosis

Hopefully what should be clear by now is that you should consider ADRs as part of the differential diagnosis of any newly presented condition. You should look out for drug-induced effects – drugs causing ADRs that might be mistaken for the symptoms of a new condition.

The following activities are designed to make you think about ADRs as part of your diagnosis. Try each, using the BNF, electronic BNF or App to assist you when necessary. Make a note of your answers before you check them against the answers given below so you can test and reinforce your own knowledge.

ACTIVITY 8.4

An 82-year-old woman has arrived at Accident & Emergency by ambulance, having collapsed in the supermarket.

Her past medical history is hypertension and angina.

Her current medications are amlodipine 5mg one daily, bendroflumethiazide 2.5mg daily, isosorbide mononitrate 20mg each morning and lunchtime, prednisolone 2.5mg one daily, alendronic acid 70mg once weekly, and Adcal D3 two daily.

Which of her drugs could have contributed to her presenting complaint?

There may be many reasons for this woman's collapse but postural hypotension is a common side-effect of isosorbide mononitrate and bendroflumethiazide and needs to be considered as part of the overall diagnosis. Note that, in the BNF, when you look up the side-effects of isosorbide mononitrate, you are guided to side-effects under glyceryl trinitrate. The side-effects are shown in the order of their frequency, so postural hypotension is the most common. For bendroflumethiazide it has also been reported frequently.

ACTIVITY 8.5 COMMON ADVERSE DRUG REACTIONS 1

A 67-year-old man has been prescribed dihydrocodeine 30mg every 4 hours for mild to moderate joint pain. Which two of the following potential ADRs are most likely to be caused by the drug?

- Sweating
- Rash
- Constipation
- Hypotension
- Nausea and vomiting

From the BNF, the most common ADRs from this list are nausea and vomiting, and constipation.

ACTIVITY 8.6 COMMON ADVERSE DRUG REACTIONS 2

A 65-year-old patient has recently had a blood test which indicates hepatic toxicity. Which one of the following drugs is most likely to be associated with this?

- Ibuprofen
- Leflunomide
- Perindopril
- Paracetamol

From the BNF you can see that leflunomide can cause potentially life-threatening hepatoxicity, usually in the first 6 months, which is why monitoring liver function is essential. In liver dysfunction, monitoring is also required when taking perindopril.

How do you know if the symptoms identified are an ADR?

Activities 8.4–8.6 have hopefully reiterated the point that symptoms being treated could be an ADR of another drug. As we said earlier, the best way to become aware of the possibility that a symptom might be an ADR, rather than evidence of a new condition, is always to consider an ADR in your differential diagnosis. We now look at how you can try to decide if a presenting symptom might be an ADR perhaps before deciding on a Yellow Card Scheme report or a change in patient treatment.

As far as reporting is concerned, a suspicion is all that's needed. However, there are various ways you can try to decide if an ADR is the cause of a patient's symptoms (see Table 8.3).

Table 8.3 How to decide if an adverse drug reaction may be the cause of a patient's symptoms

Time	How long after the patient started taking the drug did he or she begin to identify symptoms?
Improvement	Did the patient improve once the drug was stopped?
Independent evidence	Is there any published evidence that shows the patient's symptoms could be drug-induced?
Predictability	Has this reaction been reported before, or could it be predicted based on the known properties of the drug?

All these factors would suggest causality. However, nothing is absolute and it is not always easy to predict. The important thing is to consider it and if a drug can be changed and symptoms may be related to the drug, it is sensible to consider the change.

How can you reduce the risk of adverse drug reactions?

Knowing the type of patients or conditions that might predispose a patient to suffer an ADR and knowing the types of drug that cause most ADRs will help you when you are prescribing. Make sure the dose and drug choice are appropriate for the age of the patient. Always discuss the possibility of side-effects with patients and listen and react to their concerns. If patients decide to continue treatment, ensure they receive counselling on the correct use of medicines and what to do if they do suspect side-effects. Barry *et al.* (2000) suggest that wanting to know about possible side-effects is often part of an unvoiced agenda patients have at the consultation. In addition:

- Always take or refer to a detailed drug history when starting a new drug, including any previous ADRs.
- Only use drug treatments when there is a clear indication.
- Stop drugs that are no longer necessary.
- Check the dose and response, especially in the young, elderly and those with renal, hepatic or cardiac disease.

Before you prescribe:

- Ensure the patient understands the likely benefits of the medication but also the risks associated. You could use patient information leaflets to inform your discussions. These can be accessed on www.medicines.org.uk.

Patients may not be aware that the generic drug they are being given by you is the same as the brand drug they got some years ago and reacted badly to. People forget!

How do you report adverse drug reactions?

The main method of postmarketing surveillance in the UK is the Yellow Card Scheme, which was started in 1964 (post thalidomide). Reports are accepted from doctors, dentists, coroners, industry, pharmacists, nurses, midwives and health visitors. Recent additions include radiographers, optometrists and patients.

The MHRA website has a useful question and answer page.

The Yellow Card Scheme has had a major impact on the labelling, warnings and availability of drugs following investigation of reports of suspected ADRs. Drugs can be withdrawn, although this is more often as a result of the pharmaceutical company removing the drug from the market voluntarily.

You can find out more about how drug surveillance and Yellow Card reports are used to develop knowledge about safe use of drugs by signing up on the MHRA website to receive its monthly drug safety update.

Looking at adverse drug reaction reports

To see if a drug you use has had ADRs reported you can use the MHRA website, www.medicines.org.uk. The reports are called DAPs. Following up the varenicline example in Activity 8.2, Figure 8.1 shows what the varenicline DAP looks like.

Drug Analysis Print
Drug name: VARENICLINE
Jump to firsr report page

Drug name:	VARENICLINE	Report type:	Spontaneous
Report run date:	29-Nov-2011	Report origin:	UNITED KINGDOM
Data lock date:	28-Nov-2011 08:00:04PM	Route of admin:	ALL
Period covered:	01-Jul-1963 to 28-Nov-2011	Reporter type:	ALL
Earliest reaction date:	26-Dec-2006	Reaction:	ALL
MedDRA version:	MedDRA 14.1	Age group:	ALL

Total number of reactions*: 18388	Total number of ADR reports: 7290	Total number of fatal ADR reports: 81

Products included in this print – Single active constituent products (PBGs):
CHAMPIX

Figure 8.1 Drug analysis print. (Reproduced with kind permission of MHRA.)

*It is important to note that one report may contain one or more reactions.

The earliest report for varenicline was in December 2006. From that date to the end of November 2011, there were over 7,000 individual reports containing over 18,000 potential ADRs with 81 deaths. The report does not prove causality and there may have been more than one drug being taken at the time and we do not know the patient's medical condition.

The process for reporting an adverse drug reaction

The process should be simple if it is to encourage more reports. If you have a BNF there is a form at the back (Figure 8.2), but many people find it is simpler to complete one online at http://yellowcard.mhra.gov.uk. You need to register once.

Think about a patient who has come in complaining of new symptoms following the prescription you gave of a newly marketed drug. After questioning you suspect that this is an adverse reaction to the drug and are considering reporting it. What should you do?

Firstly, you do not have to prove causality; a suspicion is all that is necessary, particularly for a new drug. If the drug has an inverted triangle next to it in the BNF, which shows it is new and under particular surveillance, you should report any suspected ADR. It doesn't matter how inconsequential you think the effect is, as this reporting helps build up a postmarketing picture of the new drug.

Secondly, report any serious ADR (see the definition earlier in this chapter), however established the drug is or for however long it has been on the market. The

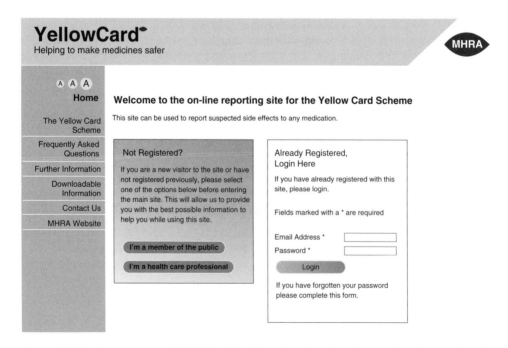

Figure 8.2 Registration page for Yellow Card for reporting drug interactions. (Reproduced with kind permission of MHRA.)

reason the MHRA continues to request reports for established drugs is because they may highlight previously unrecognised effects. For example, Reye's syndrome was associated with aspirin eight decades after it was first marketed.

Sending the report may allow advice to be given on risk factors for patients, such as age or concurrent disease, or how medicines can be used more safely. It cannot be stressed enough how important completing the Yellow Card Scheme forms can be.

Not everyone who is made aware of an adverse reaction to a drug reports it. Why do you think this is? Some suggestions for this are: complacency – a belief that only 'safe drugs' get on the market; a fear that you will be involved in litigation; guilt at prescribing the drug that caused the patient discomfort or harm; ambition to collect a series of cases before reporting; ignorance of how/what to report; fear of reporting a mere suspicion; lethargy – lack of interest or time.

Make sure this isn't you.

How might reporting be improved?

There is a need to improve both professional and public education about the Yellow Card Scheme. The use of electronic reporting is a great advance in simplifying access to reporting facilities, as are the pages in the BNF. You might consider that all healthcare professionals should be involved in reporting and this is improving. Developing an understanding by public advertising and ensuring it is part of the curriculum for all healthcare professionals who deal with medicines and patients might also help.

Chapter summary

In this chapter we discussed definitions and classifications of ADRs, including their prevalence and potential outcomes. We also briefly considered patient groups which may be more susceptible to ADRs and drug groups that cause most ADRs. ADRs are important and lead to a number of potential adverse outcomes. On the one hand it may be that the patient's view of you as the prescriber is diminished and on the other the patient may suffer harm, including death. Vigilance is essential to try to avoid ADRs and it is important to remember that any reported symptoms might be the result of an ADR to a prescribed medicine and this should be part of the differential diagnosis.

Finally we discussed how to report ADRs to improve market surveillance, particularly of new products.

Your goal is to ensure ADRs are kept to a minimum by knowing which type of drugs and which patient groups you should be particularly cautious about and, if ADRs happen, knowing how to report them.

GOING FURTHER

British Medical Journal (publisher)
   The BMJ has regular case reports which can often alert you to ADRs in a timely manner.

Davies DM, Ferner RE and de Glanville H (1998) *Davies's Textbook of Adverse Drug Reactions*, 5th edn. London: Chapman and Hall Medical.
This is a standard textbook, well laid out and comprehensive. However it is expensive and the 1998 edition is the latest.

Lee A (ed.) (2006) *Adverse Drug Reactions*, 2nd edn. London: Pharmaceutical Press.
This is a more reasonably priced, very well-written and well-laid-out book. It is fully referenced, with an excellent chapter on pharmacogenetics and adverse drug reactions related to this.

Medicines and Healthcare Products Regulatory Agency (MHRA): www.mhra.gov.uk
The MHRA website, which has been referred to throughout this chapter, is a very useful source of practical information about ADRs and how to report them.

MHRA Drug Safety Update: http://www.mhra.gov.uk/Safetyinformation/ DrugSafetyUpdate/index.htm
This is a monthly newsletter from the MHRA, covering issues around medicines use. Subscribe (free) for automatic updates.

The Medicines Information Unit of your local hospital and, of course, the British National Formulary will also be useful sources of information.

chapter 9

Drug Interactions

Barry Strickland-Hodge

Achieving your medical degree

This chapter will help you begin to meet the following requirements of *Tomorrow's Doctors* (General Medical Council (GMC), 2009):

8. (f) Demonstrate knowledge of drug actions: therapeutics and pharmacokinetics; drug side effects and interactions, including for multiple treatments, long-term conditions and non-prescribed medication; and also including effects on the population, such as the spread of antibiotic resistance.

17. Prescribe drugs safely, effectively and economically.

   (c) Provide a safe and legal prescription.

   (f) Access reliable information about medicines.

   (h) Demonstrate awareness that many patients use complementary and alternative therapies, and awareness of the existence and range of these therapies, why patients use them, and how this might affect other types of treatment that patients are receiving.

It will also link to:

Good Medical Practice (GMC, 2013a)

and

Good Practice in Prescribing and Managing Medicines and Devices (GMC, 2013b), particularly paragraphs 6–11, 24, 28 and 45.

Chapter overview

Drugs can interact with other drugs, food, herbs and biochemical tests (Baxter and Preston, 2013). Interactions can prevent one drug being absorbed or distributed around the body. They can speed up or inhibit metabolism or they can prevent or enhance elimination. Most are therefore pharmacokinetic in nature. Finally drug interactions can cause patients harm and therefore need to be considered each time you prescribe.

By reading this chapter you should be able to:

- describe what drug interactions are and how often they occur;
- use the *British National Formulary* (BNF) as a guide to drug interactions;
- recognise the main types and mechanisms of drug interactions;
- identify patients who are more susceptible and certain drugs which are more 'reactive';
- apply strategies to avoid drug interactions.

What do you think of as a drug interaction?

The BNF says:

> *Two or more drugs given at the same time may exert their effects independently or may interact. The interaction may be potentiation or antagonism of one drug by another or occasionally some other effect.*
>
> (BNF, 2012, p. 841)

Stockley, the recognised authority on interactions, gives a more succinct definition in its ninth edition:

> *a drug interaction is said to occur when the effects of one drug are changed by the presence of another drug, herbal medicine, food, drink or by some other environmental chemical agent.*
>
> (Baxter and Preston, 2013, p. 1)

The effects of one drug on another can be to enhance its effect, potentially leading to toxic levels, or it might prevent its absorption and reduce its activity. In this chapter we will look at the different types of drug interaction and make you more aware of how to reduce their impact or eliminate them altogether.

ACTIVITY 9.1 KEEPING UP TO DATE

How do you currently monitor or identify drug interactions?

Discuss this with a colleague and compare how you both deal with this potential issue.

You may have said you don't currently look for drug interactions but assume the computer or the pharmacy will spot any major ones. You might currently rely on the hospital or community pharmacists to identify drug interactions and contact you about them. You might use the BNF – we'll discuss that in a moment. If you are very fortunate you might have a copy of *Stockley's Drug Interactions* (Baxter and Preston, 2013) or the *Stockley Pocket Companion* (Baxter, 2012) to hand.

Whatever your response, if the watchwords for adverse drug reactions (ADRs: Chapter 8) are 'Always consider an ADR as part of your differential diagnosis'; then similarly with drug interactions. Always consider side-effects or new symptoms as possibly the result of a drug interaction.

What is the incidence of drug interactions?

As with ADRs (see Chapter 8), there have been various studies looking at the incidence of drug interactions. However, a number of interactions occur with a prescribed drug and something the patient may have bought or borrowed from a neighbour. They may also occur between a prescribed drug and a herbal medicine the patient has bought, or a food or drink such as grapefruit, cranberry juice or alcohol. These would be difficult to pick up in any study (Penzak, 2010). The estimates for the incidence of drug interactions relate in many ways to the number of medicines a patient is taking – polypharmacy.

Some interaction studies have been carried out without critically analysing the outcome of the interaction, so some had no clinical significance but were included. Some interactions are good if it means you can take a lower dose of one medicine by taking a second one. It has been suggested that some patients will suffer an interaction with two drugs when another patient will not (Baxter and Preston, 2013). Overall it's a much less clear picture than with ADRs (see Chapter 8).

Drug interactions may be of little clinical significance but others can be a cause of serious harm and even death. We will mention some particularly 'reactive' drugs which you need to be especially cautious about. Remember too, patients may buy potent medicines over the counter and may see more than one prescriber while taking their medication.

Where do you go for information about drug interactions?

Using the BNF as a guide

Whether you use the electronic version of the BNF, an App on your phone or the hard copy, the place to look for drug interactions is Appendix 1 of the BNF.

ACTIVITY 9.2 USING THE BNF

Look at a current edition of the hard-copy version of the BNF and find Appendix 1.

Look at any drug you are familiar with and see what it says. If the drug is listed (not all are), it may have a list of drugs in alphabetical order shown underneath it and some may have a black dot next to them. What do you think this black dot means?

If you check the introductory page of Appendix 1 you'll see that this means the interaction is potentially serious. It is a guide for you to make clinical decisions. Lists of interactions in Appendix 1 which do not have a black dot have been reviewed but there is little evidence of patient harm, although you as the prescriber are asked to be aware and make a clinical decision about risk and benefit.

The BNF is an excellent source but sometimes you need to put some work in to find exactly what you want. To take a simple example: Is there a drug interaction between phenelzine, a monoamine oxidase inhibitor (MAOI), and pseudoephedrine? Use Appendix 1 of the BNF. You can look up either drug but start with phenelzine this time. Appendix 1 is in alphabetical order and it says phenelzine – see MAOIs. Using the same Appendix, go to the section headed MAOI. All drugs in this section are listed alphabetically and you can see there are a number of drugs with black dots, indicating co-administration would lead to a potentially serious interaction. The word pseudoephedrine is not, however, in the list. Look up the word pseudoephedrine in Appendix 1 and you will be guided to sympathomimetics. Return to the section on MAOIs. In the alphabetical list in Appendix 1 you can see that there is a listing for sympathomimetics and the drug pseudoephedrine is there with a black dot. So the answer to the question 'is there a drug interaction?' is yes and it is potentially serious, leading to hypertensive crisis. This illustrates how useful the BNF is but sometimes you, the user, must use some initiative.

What are the main types of drug interaction?

The main types of drug interaction are pharmacokinetic in that one drug can affect the absorption, distribution, metabolism or excretion of another. In the less common pharmacodynamic interactions, a second drug can affect the way the first drug acts, for example, on receptors.

The most common, clinically significant pharmacokinetic drug interactions relate to metabolism. In a book of this type we will not be going into the exact mechanisms of the interactions but some pharmacology is required to understand how these interactions may happen and how they may be avoided.

Pharmacokinetic drug interactions

Absorption

The amount of drug absorbed and the speed at which it is absorbed can be affected by other drugs. One drug may speed gastric emptying which, as most drugs are absorbed in the small intestine, may speed up its absorption and therefore potentially its action. Metoclopramide increases gut motility and, if taken with paracetamol, will speed the passage of the analgesic from the stomach to the intestine, where it is absorbed, potentially leading to a faster action. This is shown in the BNF Appendix 1 as an interaction (listed under analgesics), but it's a positive one and the combination product is available for sale as a single unit. However, increasing gut motility may also have the effect of decreasing the absorption of digoxin from tablets, with more being excreted in the faeces (Manninen *et al.*, 1973). The clinical significance of this is mentioned in Baxter and Preston (2013) but is not listed in the BNF as potentially serious. This suggests you need caution to make a clinical decision based on risk–benefit and you may need to contact medicines information for further advice. Drugs such as antacids slow or prevent the absorption of, for example, ciprofloxacin by forming an insoluble chelate.

Distribution

The next pharmacokinetic element to consider is distribution. After the first drug has been absorbed, some is distributed around the body attached to proteins in the plasma. You will remember that only free drug can have an action at receptors. If a second drug competes for the binding sites on the plasma proteins, it can displace the first drug, leading to an increased concentration of free drug able to act. In the past this was thought to be of major significance. However, as the drug is displaced into the plasma it is quickly metabolised. Drug still attached to the protein is then released to create equilibrium in the plasma. It is difficult to identify any clinically significant drug interactions specifically due to plasma protein displacement. It may be important in therapeutic drug monitoring, for example with phenytoin and in some cases where the drug is given intravenously.

Metabolism

A much more important aspect of pharmacokinetic drug interactions involves metabolism in the liver and in particular the cytochrome P450 isoenzymes (of which there are more than 50). Some drugs will only be affected by specific cytochrome P450 isoenzymes and not others.

Drugs are mainly, but not exclusively, metabolised in the liver. A second drug might have the effect of inducing or inhibiting liver enzymes. Those that induce enzymes will cause the breakdown of the first drug to occur more rapidly. Consider the effect of an enzyme inducer such as rifampicin on a substrate, for example ciclosporin. The antirejection effect of ciclosporin will be reduced and therefore the potential for organ rejection is increased. Another example is the effect of rifampicin on oral contraceptives. This can lead to a failure of the contraceptive so additional contraceptive advice will be required. Drugs that inhibit the cytochrome P450 isoenzymes such as clarithromycin will have the effect of reducing the metabolism of the first drug, say ciclosporin, leading to an increase in plasma concentration of the ciclosporin and potential toxicity.

> ## Scenario 9.1: Identifying drug interactions
>
> A 20-year-old woman with epilepsy is requesting oral contraception. After undertaking the usual medical history and examination you consider prescribing Microgynon. Her notes show she is currently taking carbamazepine. Is there a problem with this combination?

In the BNF Appendix 1, Microgynon is not listed and there is no guidance as to where to look. You are expected to look under 'contraceptives, oral'. In the hard-copy BNF you will be directed to oestrogens and progestogens. These are listed separately. Under oestrogens, carbamazepine doesn't have a separate entry but antiepileptics do and, in this section, carbamazepine is shown with a black dot, where it states that metabolism of oestrogen (or progestogen) is accelerated. You are then guided to a separate section of the BNF to show what is recommended if the drugs are given together. As you can see, using the hard-copy BNF is not as straightforward as you may have hoped. In Appendix 1, carbamazepine is listed and oestrogens and progestogens are shown in the alphabetical list. So it sometimes depends on where you start your search.

Elimination

Many drugs and their metabolites are excreted by the kidney. If drugs are to be reabsorbed in the kidney tubules, they need to be in an un-ionised lipid-soluble form. If the pH of the urine is changed by another drug or food, leading to a greater degree of ionisation, there can be changes in reabsorption and therefore elimination. Weakly acidic drugs will exist in a mainly ionised (thus non-lipid-soluble) form if the urine is alkaline. They will not be reabsorbed and will therefore be eliminated in the urine. The clearance of weak bases is greater in acidic urine.

Interactions involving P-glycoprotein (P-gp) transporters

This is the last pharmacology section but it is important to understand how some drug interactions may actually happen. Drugs and other substances cross membranes by carrier-mediated processes. We have known for some time, for example, that vitamin B_{12} needs intrinsic factor to transport it across the gut wall. If this is absent the patient can develop pernicious anaemia. Whereas intrinsic factor can transport B_{12} into the cells, the P-gp transporters are able to remove substances from cells. They are large protein molecules found in the cells of the gut, gonads, kidneys, biliary system, brain and other organs. Interfering with this protein can prevent the elimination of drugs or harmful substances from cells and thus lead to potential toxicity. P-gp can be induced – eliminating more drug from cells – or inhibited – preventing removal of drugs and other substances. Atorvastatin is a P-gp inhibitor whereas rifampicin is a P-gp inducer.

What do you think would be the effect of the P-gp inducer rifampicin on the concentration of digoxin in cells? As an inducer, rifampicin increases the ejection of digoxin from cells into the gut, and thus to elimination, which lowers the digoxin plasma concentration. Whether this is clinically significant is not clear. More recently, it has been shown that ticagrelor, a P-gp inhibitor, can increase the plasma concentration of digoxin and ciclosporin significantly and appropriate clinical and/ or laboratory monitoring is recommended when given concomitantly (Summary of Product Characteristics, Brilique, 2011). We are continuing to find out more about these transporter proteins and therefore understand more about drug interactions.

Drug–food and drug–herb interactions

The absorption of drugs can be affected by the presence of food. For example, calcium in milk or other metals such as magnesium or aluminium in many antacids interact with the molecules of tetracycline to form an insoluble chelate. This well-known interaction can be avoided by taking the antibiotic on an empty stomach and avoiding milk or antacids for say 2 hours after taking the drug. Other drugs that form chelates with milk and antacids are bisphosphonates and ciprofloxacin. Other food can enhance absorption. For example if the drug requires an acid environment to be absorbed (as itraconazole does, for example) it would be best to take it with food.

Most medicines are absorbed in the small intestine so a drug that can reduce gastric emptying can delay passage to the small intestine and thus slow or delay absorption.

Cranberry juice is listed in the BNF Appendix 1 as something that interacts with anticoagulants. The BNF says it possibly enhances the anticoagulant effect of coumarins (warfarin), so avoid concomitant use. The evidence to support this interaction is weak but as the BNF is currently advising you to avoid, it is best to remain cautious. Grapefruit juice is another compound which has a number of listed interactions, many of them potentially serious (Dresser *et al.*, 2002).

As a prescriber you will need to be aware of this so you can advise patients accordingly. Pharmacists will add the warnings and advice to labels when the medicine is dispensed but verbal emphasis can enhance adherence.

Herbs such as St John's Wort have been known for some time to interact with the oestrogens and progestogens, but look at Appendix 1 of the BNF and find St John's Wort. As it's an abbreviation, it appears as the first drug in the S section of Appendix 1. Note that there are a large number of interacting drugs and that many have black dots, showing that they are potentially serious. Let us consider the evidence for one particular potential interaction – St John's Wort and emergency hormonal contraception.

What's the evidence? St John's Wort

The BNF states that St John's Wort should be avoided by women taking ulipristal, an oral emergency contraceptive, as the contraceptive effect is reduced. It is given a black dot and therefore it is considered potentially serious, leading to possible contraceptive failure.

In March 2012, the UK Medicines Information pharmacists group published a detailed document as a response to a frequently asked question entitled: Does St John's Wort interact with emergency hormonal contraception? (UKMi, 2012).

In response to this question, the UKMi noted that most of the available evidence regarding an interaction between St John's Wort (*Hypericum perforatum*) and hormonal contraceptives relates to women who were taking a combined oral hormonal contraceptive, not emergency hormonal contraception.

In vitro studies showed that hyperforin, a component of hypericum, is a potent inducer of the cytochrome P450 enzymes, particularly the specific isoenzyme CYP3A4, as well as affecting the P-gp transport system, mentioned earlier. However, this has not been reproduced *in vivo*. The isoenzyme CYP3A4 appears to be the major route for inactivation of most contraceptive steroids, including levonorgestrel.

UKMi summarises the findings from a 2010 pharmacokinetic study:

> *In a small pharmacokinetic study, 36 participants received either 6 weeks of placebo, herb or St John's Wort followed by the emergency hormonal contraceptive, levonorgestrel, taken between days 9–12 of a normal menstrual cycle. Serum progesterone levels were measured at weekly intervals. Pharmacokinetic modelling showed that levonorgestrel clearance increased with increasing amounts of St John's Wort. The study authors reported that the trend was consistent but not statistically significant and concluded dosing with St John's Wort may have effects on the clearance of levonorgestrel, however larger studies are needed to determine the risk of emergency contraceptive failure when using P450 enzyme inducers such as St John's Wort.*
>
> (Murphy, 2010)

As St John's Wort is an enzyme inducer, you would expect it to decrease the plasma concentration of any drug metabolised by the same isoenzyme.

UKMi also includes the advice from the Faculty of Sexual and Reproductive Healthcare (FSRH) of the Royal College of Obstetricians and Gynaecologists. In this the FSRH advises that the effectiveness of emergency hormonal contraceptives will be reduced in women taking liver enzyme inducers, including St John's Wort. Women who require emergency contraception whilst using St John's Wort or within 28 days of stopping should be advised that a copper intrauterine device is the most effective method (FSRH, 2012).

Even though the evidence is slight, the advice is to use another form of contraception (emergency or not) if the St John's Wort cannot be stopped.

In Stockley, again, the effect of St John's Wort is cited as an enzyme inducer and a P-gp inducer but the clinical significance of these actions is not so easily identified (Baxter and Preston, 2013).

What would you do and have you a system in place to identify if patients are buying medicines such as St John's Wort?

> ## Scenario 9.2
>
> Consider the case of a 40-year-old male patient who has recently undergone a kidney transplant and is receiving tacrolimus to prevent transplant rejection. When the patient leaves hospital he is naturally anxious and decides to buy St John's Wort as a mild anti-depressant. As a herb, the patient has no concern about its potency or action on the new organ or on the drugs he has been given. After all you can buy it over the counter, 'so it must be safe'.
>
> What is your reaction when you see the patient and what advice do you give?

You should be deeply concerned that this patient would take anything after such a recent transplant and while on potent medicines. However you realise that this does happen. This emphasises the importance of discussing such issues with patients and helping them to understand enough about their medication to take it safely while maintaining their confidence in the treatment and you.

You need to explain, in whatever language you feel appropriate for this patient, that taking St John's Wort can lead to transplant failure. It induces cytochrome P450 and in particular the isoenzyme CYP3A4 and this speeds up the metabolism of the antirejection drug tacrolimus. Blood levels will be significantly reduced, leading to potential rejection of the new kidney.

This interaction can occur with other enzyme inducers such as carbamazepine, phenytoin or phenobarbital, and they will cause the problem with both tacrolimus and ciclosporin.

Pharmacodynamic interactions

Pharmacodynamic interactions are less frequent than pharmacokinetic interactions, and may involve competition for receptor sites, which can be antagonistic or additive/synergistic.

An obvious example of an antagonistic interaction is a beta-blocker such as propranolol taken with salbutamol, a beta 2 agonist. The bronchodilator effects of the salbutamol are blocked by the non-specific (beta 1 and beta 2) beta-blocker. Another example in the same area would be anticoagulants interacting with vitamin K. (This can be found in Appendix 1 of the BNF under Vitamins.)

Think of an additive interaction where the effects of one drug are enhanced by another.

You may have said that any drug in the same class as another will be potentially additive and that is often the case. One simple example is the potassium-sparing diuretic spironolactone with angiotensin-converting enzyme inhibitors, which are also potassium sparing, where this can lead to hyperkalaemia. Alcohol plus any central nervous system-depressant drug can exhibit additive effects. Looking at our definition of a drug interaction, these are not strictly speaking one drug interacting with another and hence they are rarely included in the BNF, but it is important to consider them when counselling patients about their medicines.

Susceptible patients

As with ADRs, there are patient groups who may be more susceptible to drug interactions. However, unlike ADRs, they are not necessarily easy to classify. The most obvious group are those taking a number of medicines – polypharmacy – which may be unavoidable but is always worth reviewing regularly. The elderly, those with renal or hepatic disease, the seriously or chronically ill patient and those with acute illnesses but with existing serious conditions (such as those taking antirejection medication after a transplant) are all at risk. The biggest factor is polypharmacy.

Genetic factors may also play a part in the susceptibility of certain patients to drug interactions. As with ADRs, metabolism is the most likely focus. Those who are unable to metabolise one drug may be more susceptible to the actions of a second drug (for more information about specific patient groups, see Chapter 6, and for more information about ADRs, see Chapter 8).

Specific drugs

Looking at the BNF Appendix 1 again, you can see that some drugs have more black dots (potentially serious) next to drugs in the list below them than others. Look, for example, at lithium, then at MAOIs which you looked at earlier. You can see that the majority of drugs taken with lithium or the MAOIs have interactions that could be potentially serious. By contrast, metoclopramide has only one drug interaction listed (ciclosporin) as potentially serious. Have a look at drugs you commonly use in practice and see which potentially serious drug interactions are possible.

How can you avoid drug interactions?

Keeping the number of medications given to patients to a minimum is the best way. It is also crucial to understand that drugs interact with not only other drugs, but also with food and herbal remedies, which patients may be buying for themselves.

Other practical points include the following:

- The impact of an interaction will be greatest in drugs with a narrow therapeutic range. This includes phenytoin, digoxin and warfarin.
- Be aware of the pharmacology of drugs you use, to avoid the pharmacodynamic interactions.
- Take extra care in the elderly, who are likely to be on more drugs and also to have less metabolic capacity.
- Don't forget to consider interactions when stopping drugs as well as when starting them.

Chapter summary

It is impossible to remember all drug interactions but if you begin to specialise you should be able to remember the main ones in your area. Knowing how interactions can happen can help you prevent them. Polypharmacy and age are known to increase the chance of an interaction. Remember that it isn't just other drugs you or your colleagues may have prescribed for a patient but also herbs, food including fruit juices, alcohol and tobacco they may have bought. Know how to use the BNF. It looks easy but there are issues around grouping drugs in the Appendices. Look at the cautionary labels appendix as well as the interactions appendix and this can often guide you when advising patients when to take their medicines.

GOING FURTHER

Baxter K (2012) *Stockley's Drug Interactions: Pocket companion.* London: Royal Pharmaceutical Society of Great Britain.

Baxter K and Preston CL (eds) (2013) *Stockley's Drug Interactions: A source book of interactions, their mechanisms, clinical importance and management,* 10th edn. London: Pharmaceutical Press.

British National Formulary, latest edition. London: Joint Committee of the Royal Pharmaceutical Society, BMA, Pharmaceutical Press.

Brunton LL (ed.) (2006) *Goodman & Gilman's the Pharmacological Basis of Therapeutics,* 11th edn. New York: McGraw-Hill.

appendix 1

Drug Calculations

Here are ten typical situations where a dose needs to be calculated. None are too difficult. Think carefully, as it can be easy to make mistakes. The answers follow in Appendix 2 so you can check how you did.

1. The dose of tinzaparin for the treatment of pulmonary embolism is 175 units/kg. You have a patient who weighs 56kg. The tinzaparin preparation is 20,000 units/mL.

   What is the dose?

   What volume should be administered?

2. A 25kg child with tuberculosis requires the following oral medicines.

   What doses should be prescribed?

   What volumes should be administered?

Rifampicin	10mg/kg;	liquid	100mg/5mL
Isoniazid	10mg/kg;	liquid	50mg/5mL
Pyrazinamide	35mg/kg;	liquid	500mg/5mL
Ethambutol	15mg/kg;	liquid	200mg/5mL

3. A patient who is nil-by-mouth requires 200 micrograms of digoxin intravenously. You have 0.5mg in 2mL injection available.

   What volume should be administered?

4. A 62kg, 80-year-old patient requires a 5mg/kg loading dose of intravenous aminophylline for severe chronic obstructive pulmonary disease. You have 250mg in 10mL ampoules available.

   What is the dose?

   What volume is required?

5. A 68.5kg patient with pneumonia requires gentamicin 7mg/kg. You have gentamicin injection 80mg/2mL available.

   What is the dose?

   What volume of gentamicin injection is needed?

6. A 70kg patient requires intravenous lorazepam for a severe, acute panic attack at a dose of 30 micrograms/kg. You have lorazepam injection 4mg/mL available.

What is the dose?

What volume should be administered?

7. A 65kg patient is admitted with a paracetamol overdose and requires an infusion of acetylcysteine at 100mg/kg. You have ampoules of acetylcysteine 2g/10mL available. The infusion needs to be given in 1 litre of glucose 5% over 16 hours.

   What is the dose?

   What volume of acetylcysteine is needed?

   How would you prepare and administer the infusion?

8. A 70kg patient requires dopamine 4 micrograms/kg/min. The pharmacy supplies pre-made syringes containing 200mg in 50mL.

   What is the dose?

   What rate in mL/hour needs to be administered?

9. A 25kg child with severe hyperkalaemia requires salbutamol 4 micrograms/kg by intravenous injection. You have 500 micrograms/mL injection available. The injection needs to be diluted with glucose 5% to a concentration of 50 micrograms/mL prior to administration.

   What is the dose?

   How would you prepare the injection?

10. A 2.8kg neonate requires meropenem intravenous infusion 20mg/kg for septicaemia. You have meropenem 500mg injection (dry powder) available. You speak to the on-call pharmacist who says to reconstitute the meropenem with Water for Injection to make 10mL and that meropenem has a displacement value of 0.4mL. Then you need to dilute further with sodium chloride 0.9% to obtain a 10mg/mL solution.

    What is the dose?

    How would you prepare the infusion?

    What volume of meropenem 10 mg/mL needs to be administered?

appendix 2

Answers to Drug Calculations

1. Dose = 9,800 units
   Volume = 0.49mL (would round up to 0.5mL)

2. Rifampicin   250mg; 12.5mL of 100mg/5mL
   Isoniazid   250mg; 25mL of 50mg/5mL
   Pyrazinamide   875 mg; 8.75mL of 500mg/5ml
   Ethambutol   375mg; 9.4mL of 200mg/5mL

3. Volume = 0.5mg in 2mL ≡ 500 micrograms in 2mL
   200 micrograms ÷ 500 micrograms × 2mL = 0.8mL

4. Dose = 62 kg × 5mg = 310mg
   Volume = 310mg ÷ 250mg × 10mL = 12.4mL

5. Dose = 68.5kg × 7mg = 479.5mg (round up to 480mg)
   Volume needed = 480mg ÷ 80mg × 2mL = 12mL

6. Dose = 70kg × 30 micrograms = 2100 micrograms, 2100 micrograms ÷ 1000 = 2.1mg
   Volume = 2.1mg ÷ 4mg × 1mL = 0.53mL

7. Dose = 65 kg × 100 mg = 6500mg ≡ 6.5g
   Volume of acetylcysteine = 6.5g ÷ 2g × 10ml = 32.5mL
   Preparation/administration = remove 32.5mL from 1L glucose 5% bag and add 32.5mL acetylcysteine 2g/10mL. Run the infusion at 62.5mL/hour (1000mL ÷ 16).

8. Rate = 4 micrograms/kg/min = 4 × 70kg micrograms/min = 280 micrograms/min
   Want rate per hour so 280 micrograms/min = 280 × 60 micrograms/hour
   = 16800 micrograms/hour
   = 16800 ÷ 1000
   = 16.8 mg/hour
   Have 200mg in 50mL, want 16.8mg/hour so (16.8mg ÷ 200mg) × 50mL = 4.2 ml/hour

9. Dose = 100 micrograms (25 kg × 4 micrograms)
   100 micrograms ÷ 500 micrograms × 1mL = 0.2mL of injection needed

10. Dose = 20mg × 2.8kg = 56mg
    Infusion preparation = add 9.6mL Water for Injection to the 500mg vial of mero-penem. This gives 500mg in 10mL (as displacement value is 0.4mL) i.e. 50mg/mL. Therefore, this needs diluting by a factor of five to obtain a 10mg/mL solution.

    Take 10mL of the 500mg/10mL solution and add to 40mL of sodium chloride 0.9% . This gives 500mg in 50mL i.e. 10mg/mL

    Need 56mg dose, so 56mg ÷ 10 mg × 1mL = 5.6mL

    Give 5.6 mL over 15–30 minutes. (Could also give over 5 minutes as bolus.)

References

Alldred DP, Barber N, Buckle P *et al.* (2008) *Medication Errors in Nursing and Residential Care Homes: Prevalence, consequences, causes and solutions.* Report to the Patient Safety Research Portfolio. London: Department of Health.

Anderson G (2005) Pregnancy induced changes in pharmacokinetics: A mechanistic-based approach. *Clinical Pharmacokinetics*, 44: 989–1008.

Aronson JK (2009) Medication errors: Definitions and classification. *British Journal of Clinical Pharmacology*, 67 (6): 599–604.

Audit Office (1994) *A Prescription for Improvement: Towards more rational prescribing in general practice.* London: HMSO.

Baglin T, Cousins D, Keeling D, Perry D and Watson H (2006) Recommendations from the British Committee for Standards in Haematology and National Patient Safety Agency. *British Journal of Haematology*, 136: 26–29.

Balint M, Hunt J, Joyce D *et al.* (1970) *Treatment or Diagnosis: A study of repeat prescriptions in general practice.* London: Tavistock.

Bandolier (1997) *NNTs for Stroke Prevention.* Available online at: www.medicine.ox.ac.uk/bandolier/band38/b38-2.html (accessed 24 October 2012).

Barber N (1995) What constitutes good prescribing? *British Medical Journal*, 310: 923–925.

Barber ND, Alldred DP, Raynor DK *et al.* (2009) Care homes' use of medicines study: Prevalence, causes and potential harm of medication errors in care homes for older people. *Quality and Safety in Health Care*, 18: 341–346.

Barofsky I (1978) Compliance, adherence and therapeutic alliance: Steps in the development of self-care. *Social Science and Medicine*, 12 (5): 369–376.

Barry C, Bradley CP, Britten N *et al.* (2000) Patients' unvoiced agendas in general practice consultations: Qualitative study. *British Medical Journal*, 320: 1246.

Baxter K (ed.) (2010) *Stockley's Drug Interactions: A source book of interactions, their mechanisms, clinical importance and management*, 9th edn. London: Pharmaceutical Press.

Baxter K (2012) *Stockley's Drug Interactions: Pocket companion.* London: Royal Pharmaceutical Society of Great Britain.

Baxter K and Preston CL (eds) (2013) *Stockley's Drug Interactions: A source book of interactions, their mechanisms, clinical importance and management*, 10th edn. London: Pharmaceutical Press.

Berlin A and Carter F (2007) Using the clinical consultation as a learning opportunity. Available online at: http://www.faculty.londondeanery.ac.uk/e-learning/feedback/files/Using_the_clinical_consultation_as_a_learning_opportunity.pdf (accessed August 2013).

Birks Y and Watt I (2007) Emotional intelligence and patient-centred care. *Journal of the Royal Society of Medicine*, 100: 369–374.

Black N (1996) Why we need observational studies to evaluate the effectiveness of health care. *British Medical Journal*, 312: 1215–1218.

Bombay hospital motto. Adapted from a quotation of Mahatma Gandhi. Available online at: http://dignifiedrevolution.org.uk/about-us/background-information.html (accessed 11 July 2012).

Bond C (2001) Pharmacists and the multi-disciplinary health care team. In: Taylor K and Harding G (eds) *Pharmacy Practice.* London: Taylor and Francis, pp. 254–255.

British National Formulary (2012) Number 63, Appendix 1: Drug interactions. London: Joint Committee of the Royal Pharmaceutical Society, BMA, Pharmaceutical Press.

British National Formulary (2013) London: Joint Committee of the Royal Pharmaceutical Society, BMA, Pharmaceutical Press.

Bub B (2004) The patient's lament: Hidden key to effective communication: How to recognise and transform. *Medical Humanities*, 30: 63–69.

CAIPE (2002) Definition of IPE. Available online at: www.caipe.org.uk/about-us/defining-ipe (accessed 16 June 2012).

Cancer Research UK Smoking Statistics. Available online at: http://info.cancerresearchuk.org/cancerstats/types/lung/smoking

Cox K, Britten N, Hooper R and White P (2007) Patient involvement in decisions about medicines: GPs' perceptions of their preferences. *British Journal of General Practice*, 57: 777–784.

Croskerry P (2009) Context is everything or how could I have been that stupid? *Healthcare Quarterly*, 12 (special issue): 171–176.

Dean B, Barber N and Schachter M (2000) What is a prescribing error? *Quality in Health Care*, 9: 232–237.

Dean B, Schachter M, Vincent C and Barber N (2002) Causes of prescribing errors in hospital inpatients: A prospective study. *Lancet*, 359 (9315): 1373–1378.

Department of Health (1998) *Review of Prescribing, Supply and Administration of Medicines: A report on the supply and administration of medicines under group protocols.* London: Department of Health.

Department of Health (1999) *Making a Difference: Strengthening the nursing, midwifery and health visitor contribution to health and healthcare.* London:

Department of Health. Available online at: http://webarchive.nationalarchives.gov.uk/+/www.dh.gov.uk/en/Publicationsandstatistics/Publications/PublicationsPolicyAndGuidance/DH_4007599 (accessed August 2013).

Department of Health (2000a) *The NHS Plan: A plan for investment, a plan for reform.* London: Department of Health. Available online at: http://webarchive.nationalarchives.gov.uk/+/www.dh.gov.uk/en/publicationsandstatistics/publications/publicationspolicyandguidance/dh_4002960 (accessed August 2013).

Department of Health (2000b) *Pharmacy in the Future: Implementing the NHS plan.* London: Department of Health. Available online at: http://webarchive.nationalarchives.gov.uk/+/www.dh.gov.uk/en/Publicationsandstatistics/Publications/AnnualReports/Browsable/DH_4989549 (accessed August 2013).

Department of Health (2000c) *Patient Group Directions.* HSC 2000/026. London: Department of Health.

Department of Health (2001) *Medicines and Older People: Implementing medicines-related aspects of the NSF for older people.* London: Department of Health.

Department of Health (2003) *Winning Ways: Working together to reduce healthcare associated infections in England.* London: HMSO.

Department of Health (2004) *National Service Framework for Children, Young People and Maternity Services: Medicines for children and young people.* London: Department of Health. Available online at: www.dh.gov.uk/prod_consum_dh/groups/dh_digitalassets/@dh/@en/documents/digitalasset/dh_4090563.pdf (accessed 21 September 2012).

Department of Health (2005) *The National Service Framework for Renal Services Part Two: Chronic kidney disease, acute renal failure and end of life care.* London: Department of Health.

Department of Health (2007) *Management of Medicines: A resource to support implementation of the wider aspects of medicines management for the National Service Frameworks for Diabetes Renal Services and Long-Term Conditions.* London: Department of Health.

Department of Health (2010) *Access to the NHS by Foreign Nationals: Government response to the consultation.* Available online at: http://www.dh.gov.uk/prod_consum_dh/groups/dh_digitalassets/documents/digitalasset/dh_125285.pdf (accessed 22 November 2012).

Department of Health (2011a) *Stay Smart Then Focus: Guidance for antimicrobial stewardship in hospitals (England).* London: HMSO.

Department of Health (2011b) *The 'Never Events' List 2011/12: Policy framework for use in the NHS.* Available online at: www.dh.gov.uk/en/Publicationsandstatistics/Publications/PublicationsPolicyAndGuidance/DH_124552 (accessed 22 December 2011).

Department of Health (2012) *The 'Never Events' List 2012/13: Policy framework for use in the NHS*. London: HMSO.

Derby Hospitals Foundation Trust (2012) *Drug Names That Look and Sound Alike*. Available online at: www.derbyhospitals.nhs.uk/primary-care-staff/pharmacy/formulary/drug-names-that-look-sound-alike (accessed 3 January 2012).

Deveugele M, Derese A, De Bacquer D, van den Brink-Muinen A, Bensing J and De Maeseneer J (2004) Consultation in general practice: A standard operating procedure? *Patient Education and Counselling*, 54 (2): 227–233.

DHSS (1986) *Neighborhood Nursing: A focus for care* (Cumberlege report). London: HMSO.

DiMatteo M (2004) The role of effective communication with children and their families in fostering adherence to pediatric regimens. *Patient Education and Counselling*, 55: 339–344.

Dornan T, Ashcroft D, Heathfield H *et al.* (2009) *An In Depth Investigation into Causes of Prescribing Errors by Foundation Trainees in Relation to their Medical Education*. EQUIP study. Available online at: www.gmc-uk.org/about/research/research_commissioned_4.asp (accessed 22 December 2011).

Dresser GK, Bailey DG, Leake BF *et al.* (2002) Fruit juices inhibit organic anion transporting polypeptide-mediated drug uptake to decrease the oral availability of fexofenadine. *Clinical Pharmacology and Therapeutics*, 71 (1): 11–20.

Dunagan WC, Woodward RS, Medoff G *et al.* (1989) Antimicrobial misuse in patients with positive blood cultures. *American Journal of Medicine*, 87 (3): 253–259.

Edlin G and Golanty E (1992) *Health and Wellness: A holistic approach*, 4th edn. Boston, MA: Jones & Bartlett.

Edwards IR and Aronson JK (2000) Adverse drug reactions: Definitions, diagnosis and management. *Lancet*, 356: 1255–1259.

Einarson TR, Gutierrez LM and Rudis M (1993) Drug-related hospital admissions. *Annals of Pharmacotherapy*, 27: 832–1259.

Ferner RE and Aronson JK (2006) Clarification of terminology in medication errors: Definitions and classification. *Drug Safety*, 29 (11): 1011–1022.

Franklin BD, Vincent C, Schachter M *et al.* (2005) The incidence of prescribing errors in hospital inpatients: An overview of the research methods. *Drug Safety*, 28 (10): 891–900.

Fraser R (1999) The consultation. In: Fraser R (ed.) *Clinical Method: A general practice approach*, 3rd edn. Oxford: Butterworth Heinemann, p. 34.

Faculty of Sexual and Reproductive Healthcare (2012) *Clinical Effectiveness Unit Clinical Guidance: Emergency contraception*. Available online at: http://www.fsrh.org/pdfs/CEUguidanceEmergencyContraception11.pdf (accessed August 2013).

Gabbay J and le May A (2004) Evidence based guidelines or collectively constructed 'mindlines'? Ethnographic study of knowledge management in primary care. *British Medical Journal*, 329: 1013–1017.

Gask L and Usherwood T (2002) ABC of psychological medicine: The consultation. *British Medical Journal*, 324: 1567–1569.

General Medical Council (2006) *Good Medical Practice.* Available online at: www.gmc-uk.org/guidance

General Medical Council (2009) *Tomorrow's Doctors: Education outcomes and standards for undergraduate medical education.* Available online at: www. gmc-uk.org/guidance

General Medical Council (2012) *Investigating the Prevalence and Causes of Prescribing Errors in General Practice: The PRACtICe Study.* Available online at: http://www.gmc-uk.org/Investigating_the_prevalence_and_causes_of_prescribing_errors_in_general_practice___The_PRACtICe_study_Reoprt_May_2012_48605085.pdf (accessed 21 November 2012).

General Medical Council (2013a) *Good Medical Practice.* London: General Medical Council. Available online at: www.gmc-uk.org/static/documents/content/GMP_2013.pdf_51447599.pdf (accessed 3 July 2013).

General Medical Council (2013b) *Good Practice in Prescribing and Managing Medicines and Devices.* London: General Medical Council. Available online at: www.gmc-uk.org/Prescribing_guidance_Last_ever_final_update_29_4_13.pdf_51867046.pdf (accessed 8 July 2013).

Gillard S, Benson J and Silverman J (2009) Teaching and assessment of explanation and planning in medical schools in the United Kingdom: Cross sectional questionnaire survey. *Medical Teacher*, 31 (4): 328–331.

Gillespie L, Robertson MC, Gillespie WJ *et al.* (2009) *Interventions for Preventing Falls in Older People Living in the Community.* Cochrane Database of Systematic Reviews, Issue 2.

Gittell J, Fairfield K, Bierbaum B *et al.* (2000) Impact of relational co-ordination on quality care, postoperative pain and functioning, and length of stay: A nine hospital study of surgical patients. *Medical Care*, 38: 807–819.

Gray D and Toghill P (eds) (2000) *Introduction to the Symptoms and Signs of Clinical Medicine: A hands-on guide to developing core skills.* London: Hodder Arnold.

Greenhalgh T (2012) Why do we always end up here? Evidence-based medicine's conceptual cul-de-sacs and some off-road alternative routes. *Journal of Primary Health Care*, 4: 92–97.

Greenhalgh T and Donald A (2002) *Evidence Based Medicine as a Tool for Quality Improvement.* Oxford: Oxford University Press.

Griffin SJ, Borch-Johnsen K, Davies MJ *et al.* (2011) Effect of early intensive multifactorial therapy on 5-year cardiovascular outcomes in individuals with type 2 diabetes detected by screening (ADDITION-Europe): A cluster-randomised trial. *Lancet*, 378: 156–167.

Hammick M, Freeth D, Copperman J and Goodsman D (2009) *Being Interprofessional.* Cambridge: Polity.

Harris C and Dajda R (1996) The scale of repeat prescribing. *British Journal of General Practice*, 46 (412): 649–653.

Haynes R, Taylor D and Sackett D (1979) *Compliance in Health Care.* Baltimore, MD: Johns Hopkins University Press.

Health Protection Agency (2010) *Management of Infection Guidance for Primary Care for Consultation and Local Adaptation.* London: HMSO.

Hernandez-Diaz S and Rodriguez L (2000) Association between nonsteroidal anti-inflammatory drugs and upper gastrointestinal tract bleeding/perforation: An overview of epidemiologic studies published in the 1990s. *Archives of Internal Medicine*, 160 (14): 2093–2099.

Horne R, Weinman J, Barber N, Elliott R and Morgan M (2005) *Concordance, Adherence and Compliance in Medicine Taking: Report for the National Co-ordinating Centre for NHS Service Delivery and Organisation R & D (NCCSDO).* Available online at: http://www.netscc. ac.uk/hsdr/files/project/SDO_FR_08-1412-076_V01.pdf (accessed 28 August 2013).

Kafka F (1983) *A Country Doctor: The Penguin complete short stories of Franz Kafka* (Glatzer NN (ed.)). London: Penguin.

Keeling D, Baglin T, Tait C *et al.* (2011) Guidelines on oral anticoagulation with warfarin, 4th edn. *British Journal of Haematology*, 154 (3): 311–324.

Kurtz S, Silverman J, Benson J and Draper J (2003) Marrying content and process in clinical method teaching: Enhancing the Calgary–Cambridge guides. *Academic Medicine*, 78: 8.

Leipzig R, Cumming R and Tinetti M (1999a) Drugs and falls in older people: A systematic review and meta-analysis, Part I. Psychotropic drugs. *Journal of the American Geriatric Society*, 47: 30–39.

Leipzig R, Cumming R and Tinetti M (1999b) Drugs and falls in older people: A systematic review and meta-analysis, Part II. Cardiac and analgesic drugs. *Journal of the American Geriatric Society*, 47: 40–50.

Lewis P, Dornan T, Taylor D, Tully M, Wass V and Ashcroft D (2009) Prevalence, incidence and nature of prescribing errors in hospital inpatients. *Drug Safety*, 32: 379–389.

Lindeman R (1992) Changes in renal function with aging: Implications for treatment. *Drugs and Aging*, 2 (5): 423–431.

Mangoni A and Jackson S (2003) Age-related changes in pharmacokinetics and pharmacodynamics: Basic principles and practical applications. *British Journal of Clinical Pharmacology,* 57: 6–14.

Manninen V, Melin J, Apajalahti A and Karesoja M (1973) Altered absorption of digoxin in patients given propantheline and metoclopramide. *Lancet,* 301 (7800): 398–400. Available online at: http://www.sciencedirect.com/science/article/pii/S0140673673902523 (accessed 23 July 2012).

Marinker M (1997) *From Compliance to Concordance: Achieving shared goals in medicine taking.* London: Royal Pharmaceutical Society of Great Britain.

Marshall M and Bibby J (2011) Supporting patients to make the best decisions. *British Medical Journal,* 342: d2117.

Maskrey N, Hutchinson A and Underhill J (2009a) Getting a better grip on research: The comfort of opinion. *InnovAiT,* 2: 679–686.

Maskrey N, Underhill J, Hutchinson A *et al.* (2009b) Getting a better grip on research: A simple system that works. *InnovAiT,* 2: 739–749.

Mason JK and Laurie GT (2011) *Mason & McCall-Smith's Law and Medical Ethics,* 8th edn. Oxford: Oxford University Press.

McDowell SE, Coleman JJ and Ferner RE (2006) Systematic review and meta-analysis of ethnic differences in risks of adverse reactions to drugs used in cardiovascular medicine. *British Medical Journal,* 332 (7551): 1177–1181.

McDowell SE, Ferner HS and Ferner RE (2009) The pathophysiology of medication errors: How and where they arise. *British Journal of Clinical Pharmacology,* 67 (6): 605–613.

Medusa Injectable Medicines Guide. Southern Health NHS Foundation Trust. Available online at: http://www.southernhealth.nhs.uk/knowledge/medicines-management/medusa (accessed August 2013).

MHRA (2008) *Advice for Healthcare Professionals.* Drug Safety Update 1 (11). Available online at: www.mhra.gov.uk/Safetyinformation/index.htm

MHRA (2012) *Legal Status and Reclassification.* Available online at: www.mhra.gov.uk/Howweregulate/Medicines/Licensingofmedicines/Legalstatusandreclassification/index.htm (accessed December 2012).

Moutlon L (2007) *The Naked Consultation: A practical guide to primary care consultation skills.* Abingdon: Radcliffe.

Mowat C, Cole A, Windsor A *et al.* (2011) Guidelines for the management of inflammatory bowel disease in adults. *Gut,* 60: 571–607.

Murphy P (2010) Effects of St John's Wort on the pharmacokinetics of levonorgestrel in emergency contraceptive (EC) dosing. *Contraception,* 83: 191.

National Patient Safety Agency (2002) Patient safety alert. *Potassium Solutions: Risks to patients from errors occurring during intravenous administration.* NPSA/2002/1051. Available online at: www.npsa.nhs.uk

National Patient Safety Agency (2006a) Patient safety alert 13. *Improving Compliance with Oral Methotrexate Dosing Guidelines.* NPSA/2006/13. Available online at: www.npsa.nhs.uk

National Patient Safety Agency (2006b) *Risk Assessment of Anticoagulation Treatment.* Available online at: www.npsa.nhs.uk/health/alerts

National Patient Safety Agency (2007a) Patient safety alert 18. *Actions That Can Make Anticoagulant Therapy Safer.* NPSA/2007/18. Available online at: www.npsa.nhs.uk

National Patient Safety Agency (2007b) Safety in doses. *Improving the Use of Medicines in the NHS: Learning from national reporting.* Available online at: www.npsa.nhs.uk

National Patient Safety Agency (2008a) Rapid response report. *Reducing Dosing Errors with Opioid Medicines.* Additional supporting information. NPSA/2008/RRR005. Available online at: www.npsa.nhs.uk

National Patient Safety Agency (2008b) Rapid response report. *Risks of Incorrect Dosing of Oral Anti-cancer Medicines.* NPSA/2008/RRR001. Available online at: www.npsa.nhs.uk

National Patient Safety Agency (2009) Safety in doses. *Improving the Use of Medicines in the NHS: Learning from national reporting.* Available online at: www.npsa.nhs.uk

National Patient Safety Agency (2010a) Rapid response report. *Reducing Treatment Dose Errors with Low Molecular Weight Heparins.* NPSA/2010/RRR014. Available online at: www.npsa.nhs.uk

National Patient Safety Agency (2010b) Rapid response report. *Safer Administration of Insulin.* NPSA/2010/RRR013. Available online at: www.npsa.nhs.uk

National Patient Safety Agency (2010c) Rapid response report. *Safer Administration of Insulin. Additional supporting information.* NPSA/2010/RRR013. Available online at: www.npsa.nhs.uk

National Patient Safety Agency (2011) Rapid response report. *The Adult Patient's Passport to Safer Use of Insulin.* NPSA/2011/PSA003. Available online at: www.npsa.nhs.uk

National Prescribing Centre (2007) *A Competency Framework for Shared Decision-making with Patients: Achieving concordance for taking medicines.* Available online at: www.npc.co.uk/patients_medicines/adherence

National Prescribing Centre (2008) *Dispensing with Repeats: A practical guide to repeat dispensing,* 2nd edn. Available online at: http://www.npc.nhs.uk/

repeat_medication/repeat_dispensing/resources/dwr_for_web.pdf (accessed 16 November 2012).

National Prescribing Centre (2010) *10 Tips for GPs: Strategies for safer prescribing*. Available online at: www.npc.co.uk/evidence/top_10_tips/top_10_tips_for_GPs.php (accessed 3 January 2012).

National Prescribing Centre (2012) *A Single Competency Framework for all Prescribers*. Available online at: www.npc.co.uk/improving_quality/resources/single_comp_framework.pdf (accessed 11 October 2012).

NHS Information Centre (2012) *Prescription Cost Analysis, England 2011*. Available online at: www.ic.nhs.uk/statistics-and-data-collections/primary-care/prescriptions/prescription-cost-analysis-england--2011

NICE (2004) *Clinical Guideline 21. Falls: The assessment and prevention of falls in older people*. London: NICE.

NICE (2007) *Technical Patient Safety Solutions for Medicines Reconciliation on Admission of Adults to Hospital*. PSG001. Available online at: guidance.nice.org.uk/PSG001 (accessed 4 January 2012).

NICE (2009) *Medicines Adherence: Involving patients in decisions about prescribed medicines and supporting adherence*. Available online at: www.nice.org.uk/nicemedia/pdf/CG76FullGuideline

Nitsche CJ, Jamieson N, Lerch MM *et al.* (2010) Drug induced pancreatitis. *Best Practice & Research Clinical Gastroenterology*, 24: 143–155.

North-Lewis P (ed.) (2008) *Drugs and the Liver*. London: Pharmaceutical Press.

Oxford Dictionary (2012). Available online at: http://oxforddictionaries.com (accessed 1 July 2012).

Paediatric Formulary Committee (2013) *BNF for Children*. London: Pharmaceutical Press. Available online at: http://www.medicinescomplete.com/mc/bnfc/current (accessed August 2013).

Palliativedrugs.com. Essential independent drug information for palliative and hospice care. Available online at: http://www.palliativedrugs.com/index.html (accessed August 2013).

Patient Safety First (2008) *The How-to Guide for Reducing Harm from High Risk of Medicines*. Available online at: http://www.patientsafetyfirst.nhs.uk/ashx/Asset.ashx?path=/How-to-guides-2008-09-19/Medicines%201.1_17Sept08.pdf (accessed 28 March 2013).

Pavek P, Ceckova M and Staud F (2009) Variation of drug kinetics in pregnancy. *Current Drug Metabolism*, 10: 520–529.

Penzak SR (2010) *Drug Interactions*. Available online at: www.cc.nih.gov/training/training/principles/slides/DrugInteractions2010-2011_text.pdf (accessed July 2012).

Pharmacia Ltd (2009) *Kemicetine Succinate Injection Summary of Product Characteristics.* Available online at: www.medicines.org.uk (accessed 21 September 2012).

Picker Institute Europe (2007) *National Survey of Local Health Services 2006.* London: Department of Health.

Pietroni P (1987) Holistic medicine: New lessons to be learned. *Practitioner,* 231: 1386–1390.

Pirmohamed M, James S, Meakin S *et al.* (2004) Adverse drug reactions as a cause of admission to hospital: Prospective analysis of 18,820 patients. *British Medical Journal,* 329: 15–19.

Police Foundation (1999) *Drugs and the Law: Report of the Independent Inquiry into the Misuse of Drugs Act 1971.* Available online at: http://www.druglibrary. org/schaffer/library/studies/runciman (accessed 19 August 2013).

Pothier D, Monteiro P, Mooktiar M and Shaw A (2005) Pilot study to show the loss of important data in nursing handover. *British Journal of Nursing,* 14 (20): 1090–1093.

Power M (1998) *Working Through Communication.* Chapter 12. Listening. Available online at: http://epublications.bond.edu.au/working_through_ communication/13 (accessed 12 July 2012).

PSNC and BMA (2009) *Guidance for the Implementation of Repeat Dispensing.* Available online at: http://www.nhsemployers.org/SiteCollectionDocuments/ Repeat_dispensing_guidance_CD_090209.pdf (accessed August 2013).

Rabbi Ben Zoma (2nd century) (2006) Pirkei Avot – Ethics of the Fathers, Ch 4 V 1. *Authorised Daily Prayer Book of the United Hebrew Congregations of the Commonwealth* (Sacks J). London: Collins, p. 545.

Rawlins MD and Thompson JW (1977) Pathogenesis of adverse drug reactions. In: Davies DM (ed.) *Textbook of Adverse Drug Reactions.* Oxford: Oxford University Press, p. 44.

Reason J (1990) *Human Error.* Cambridge: University of Cambridge.

Royal Pharmaceutical Society (2011) *Keeping Patients Safe When They Transfer Between Care Providers: Getting the medicines right.* Available online at: www. rpharms.com/getting-the-medicines-right/professional-guidance.asp (accessed 3 January 2012).

Sackett DL, Rosenberg WMC, Gray JAM *et al.* (1996) Evidence based medicine: What it is and what it isn't. *British Medical Journal,* 312: 71–72.

Schaafsma F, Verbeek J, Hulshof C *et al.* (2005) Caution required when relying on a colleague's advice: A comparison between professional advice and evidence from the literature. *BMC Health Services Research,* 5: 59.

Scottish Intercollegiate Guidelines Network (2008) *Diagnosis and Management of Headaches in Adults: A national clinical guideline.* Edinburgh: Scottish

Intercollegiate Guidelines Network. Available online at: http://www.sign.ac.uk/pdf/sign107.pdf (accessed August 2013).

Shaefer C, Peters P and Miller R (eds) (2007) *Drugs During Pregnancy and Lactation*. London: Elsevier.

Shah SNH, Aslam M and Avery AJ (2001) A survey of prescription errors in general practice. *The Pharmaceutical Journal*, 267: 860–862.

Shaughnessy AF and Slawson DC (1999) Are we providing doctors with the training and tools for lifelong learning? *British Medical Journal*, 319: 1280–1282.

Shipman Inquiry Fourth Report (2004) *The Regulation of Controlled Drugs in the Community*. London: The Stationery Office.

Slawson DC and Shaughnessy AF (1997) Obtaining useful information from expert-based sources. *British Medical Journal*, 314: 947–949.

Slawson DC, Shaughnessy AF and Bennett JH (1994) Becoming an information master: Feeling good about not knowing everything. *Journal of Family Practice*, 38: 505–513.

SPC Brilique 90mg tablets (2011) *Summary of Product Characteristics*. Available online at: www.medicines.org.uk/EMC/medicine/23935/SPC/Brilique+90+mg+film+coated+tablets (accessed July 2012).

Stewart M (1995) Effective physician–patient communication and health outcomes: A review. *Canadian Medical Association Journal*, 152: 1423–1433.

The Clopidogrel in Unstable Angina to Prevent Recurrent Events (CURE) Trial Investigators (2001) Effects of clopidogrel in addition to aspirin in patients with acute coronary syndromes without ST-segment elevation. *New England Journal of Medicine*, 345: 494–502.

Thistlethwaite JE (2011) Collaboration and interprofessional working. In: McKimm J and Forrest K (eds) *Professional Practice for Foundation Doctors*. Exeter: Learning Matters, pp. 189–203.

Thistlethwaite JE and Moran M (2010) Learning outcomes for interprofessional education (IPE): Literature review and synthesis. *Journal of Interprofessional Care*, 24: 503–513.

Tuckett D, Boulton M, Olson C and Williams A (1985) *Meetings Between Experts*. London: Tavistock Publications.

Tully MP, Ashcroft DM, Dornan T *et al.* (2009) The causes of and factors associated with prescribing errors: Systematic review. *Drug Safety*, 32: 819–836.

Tunstall-Pedoe S, Rink E and Hilton S (2003) Student attitudes to undergraduate interprofessional education. *Journal of Interprofessional Care*, 17 (2): 61–172.

UCL Hospitals (2010) *Injectable Medicines Administration Guide: Pharmacy Department*, 3rd edn. London: University College London Hospitals.

UKCCC (2006) UK Council of Clinical Communication in Undergraduate Medical Education. Available online at: www.ukccc.org.uk

UKMi (2012) Medicines Q&A 34.5: *What Should You Think About When Prescribing to Pregnant Women?* National Electronic Library for Medicines. Available online at: www.nelm.nhs.uk (accessed 21 September 2012).

Vincent C (2010) *Patient Safety.* Singapore: Wiley-Blackwell.

WHO/UNICEF (2003) *Global Strategy for Infant and Young Child Feeding.* Geneva: World Health Organization.

Wiffen P, Gill M, Edwards J and Moore A (2002) Adverse drug reactions in hospital patients: A systematic review of the prospective and retrospective studies. *Bandolier Extra*, June: 1–16.

Williams S, Weinman J and Dale J (1998) Doctor–patient communication and patient satisfaction: A review. *Family Practice*, 15: 480–492.

World Health Organization (1970) International drug monitoring: The role of the hospital. A WHO report. *Drug Intelligence and Clinical Pharmacy*, 4: 101–110.

World Health Organization (2010) *Framework for Action on Interprofesssional Education and Collaborative Practice.* Geneva: WHO.

Index

In this index when referring to a group of drugs, e.g. antibiotics; anticoagulants, see also names of individual drugs e.g. penicillin; warfarin